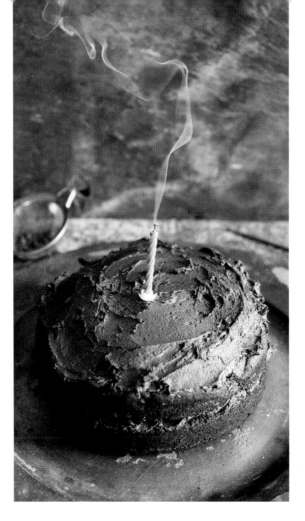

VEGAN
MAN

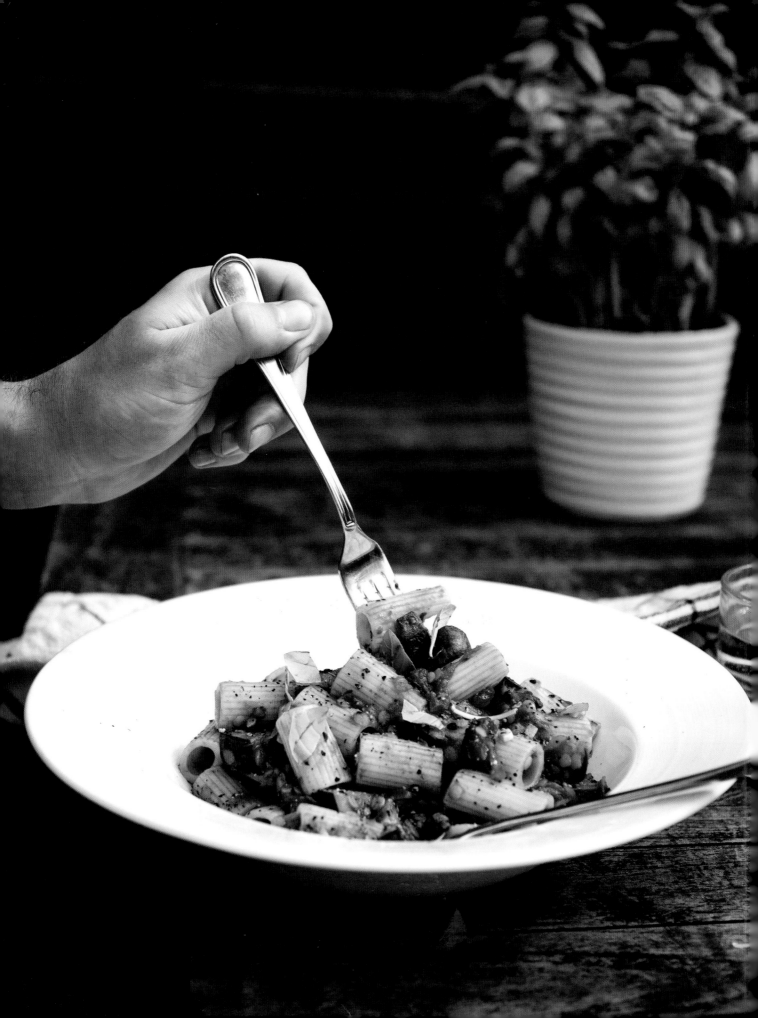

VEGAN MAN

THE MANUAL FOR COOKING AMAZING PLANT-BASED FOOD

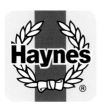

MICHAEL KITSON
FOREWORD BY JOHN ROBINS

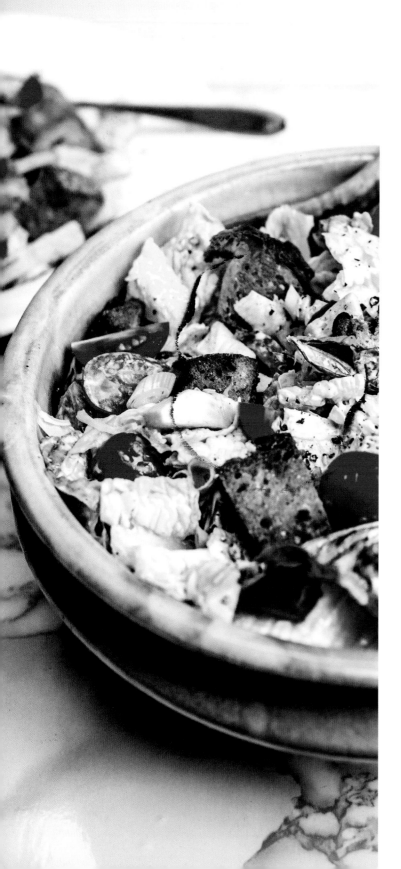

First published in 2018

A catalogue record for this book is available from the British Library.

ISBN 978 1 78521 212 3
Library of Congress control no. 2018938899

Published by Haynes Publishing,
Sparkford, Yeovil, Somerset, BA22 7JJ, UK.
Tel: 01963 440635, Int. tel: +44 1963 440635
website: www.haynes.com

Haynes North America Inc.,
859 Lawrence Drive, Newbury Park,
California 91320, USA.

Designer: Adelle Mahoney
Food photography and styling: Michael Kitson.
Additional photographs on pp 100, 103, 107, 110, 113, 114, 116, 119, 120, 129, 134, 135, 137, 139, 150 by Colin Rogal.
Images on pp10, 11, 12, 14, 15, 16, 17, 18, 19, 20, 22, 23 (bottom left) 24, 25 (top), 31 bottom, 33 supplied by Shutterstock.

Printed in Malaysia without the use of any animal-based products

ACKNOWLEDGEMENTS
Life wasn't easy when I wrote this book, and so I use this opportunity to sincerely thank and acknowledge those who helped me produce it, and to those who put me in any sort of position to be writing a book in the first place. To...

Commissioning Editor Joanne, who is the perfect combination of firm and easy-going, for her faith in me and understanding when things took an unexpected turn. Also to Colin, for his willingness, professionalism and empathy. Heather Holden-Brown, for her considerate support, and for the generosity shown to me by Matt Joblin and Becca Pusey with their professional expertise.

My father Frank, chief technical support officer and career advisor, forever devoted and supportive of my choices. My brother Tom, who only wants the best for me and has always had my back. My aunt Jack and uncle Peter, for their unquestionable or unquestioning? support and kindness. My cousin Celia, without whom my mental health would still be in pieces.

My friends Svenja, Tom, Aishlinn and best friend Sam, for their loyalty, generosity and love. Also to Teia, for her unwavering encouragement. And last but most importantly, my Mum, who plays many roles in my life, including, but not limited to, sous chef, emotional crutch, and legal advisor, without whom this book would certainly not have been finished.

CONTENTS

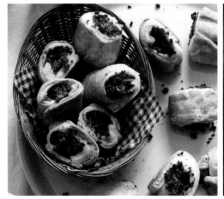 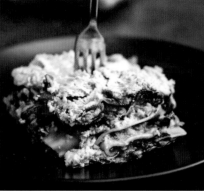 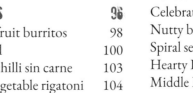

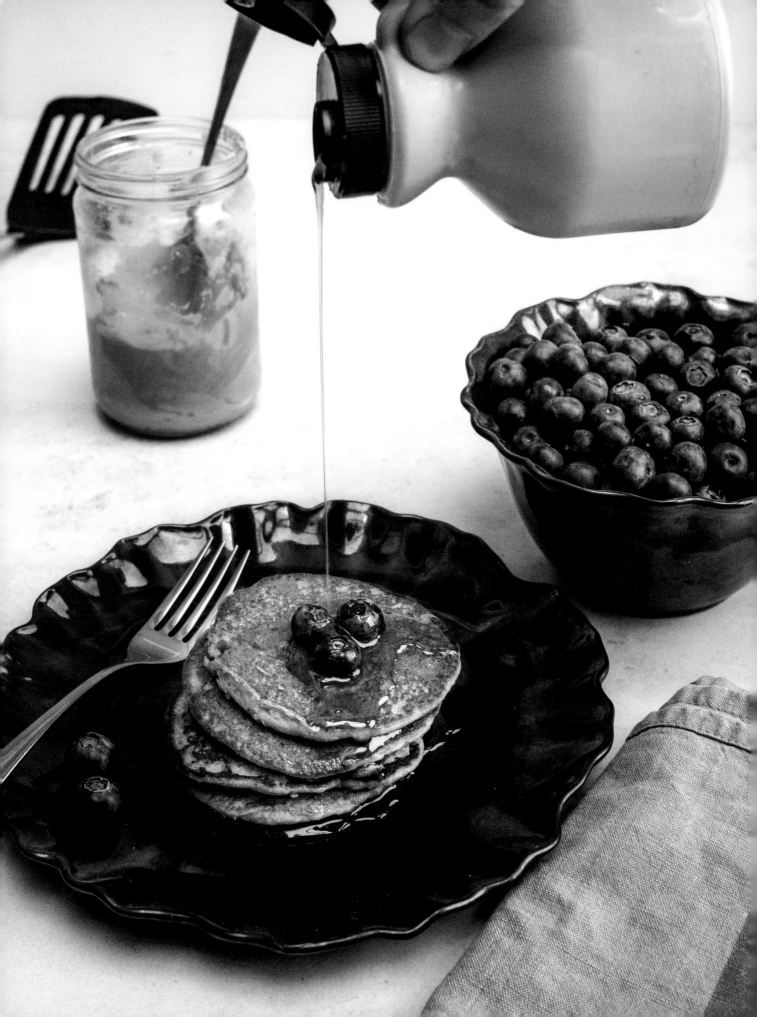

FOREWORD BY JOHN ROBINS

Hello! I am not a vegan. Well not in the strictest sense. I would describe myself as 'broadly vegan', you might describe me as a 'selective', 'flexible' or 'terrible' vegan. I first became a pescetarian about six years ago, then a vegetarian, and then, for about six months, what you might call strictly vegan. Now, about 95% of the food I eat is vegan, I'm vegan at home, but occasionally, in a poorly stocked petrol station at 2am, or when eating at a friend's house, I will let the odd splash of cheese sauce or slather of mayo slip through the net out of hunger or politeness. And I'm happy this way.

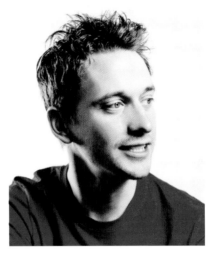

You may think I'm having my cake and eating it (I often do), but eating a vegan diet isn't a badge of honour, or a moral high ground, and the cartoon caricature of the angry, preachy vegan is something I have honestly never come across. The vegans I know chose to eat that way for many reasons, for the environment, for their health, to increase energy and concentration, but always out of kindness and empathy with animals, and horror at the way we treat them to meet the demand for huge quantities of meat and dairy products at ridiculously low prices. Eating meat more than a few times a week is a relatively recent social development, fish on a Friday and a roast joint to last the week has given way to meat on the go, sandwiches, fillings, breakfast buffets and value chicken thighs at £1.69 per kilo. Welfare at this price is not only unsustainable, it's impossible.

My vegan journey started properly in a well-known peri peri chicken restaurant. I'd been staying with a vegan for a week, and had eaten only vegan food. The experience was a revelation, at no point did I feel I was missing out, restricting myself or craving anything. That said, after leaving I headed straight for the nearest peri-peri chicken outlet and, using a full loyalty card, ordered a whole chicken. I couldn't wait. Eating it felt glorious at first, then strange, then uncomfortable. Halfway through my meal I turned the carcass over and saw something that ensured I would never eat meat again. A tumour on its ribcage. After the initial disgust subsided, I felt compassion for this chicken with cancer, 'animals get cancer?!' I thought. And at that moment, for the first time in my life, I saw the delicious meal in front of me as a living thing, something that pecked around in the dust, clucked, fancied the cockerel, slept and shat, and tried to fly. But also as a being that suffered, felt pain, got cancer. And I had got its body for free with ten stamps. And my disgust turned on myself.

We all draw lines about what we eat, ethical lines, flavour lines, lines born of squeamishness or morality. You may happily eat beef but find the idea of eating a cat despicable. You may feast on lobster but find the sight of squid vomit-inducing. You have drawn a line, a subjective, illogical, personal line that no one should ever tell you is wrong, ludicrous or inconsistent. However, one of my strongest held beliefs is that if we all ate less meat, and fewer dairy products, and spent a bit more on the meat and dairy we do eat, then the lives of the animals we rear, transport, house and slaughter would be less miserable.

Too often we only see animals in terms of their use to us. "If we didn't eat cows they wouldn't exist", is something I've heard many times from defensive meat eaters. And it's such nonsense. The mere existence of animals is a right in itself. The right to smell, to run, to fly, to mate, to hibernate, to forage, feed, gambol and interact with the world. That has such huge value in and of itself. And every time we interrupt that experience of existing, we must do so with care and with respect for that animal's right to be itself.

I used to worship meat, I was obsessed with it. But I do not miss it. When people ask me why, they often conjure up images of the perfect best-ever bacon sandwich, but how often is meat actually like that? What I don't miss is BAD MEAT. Think of all the disappointing meat you eat, the cheap sausages, the watery bacon, plastic rubbery ham in supermarket sandwiches, and reformed chicken chunks. And now imagine your favourite meat. How much of that flavour experience is nothing to do with meat at all? So much of it is the condiments and sides, mustard and ketchup, chilli sauce, mayo and gravy, all of which is vegan already or is replicated by vegan versions.

When people ask what being vegan is like, firstly, I put them straight and confess that I ate a mini baby bell at Reading Services last week, but then I'll ask what their favourite part of a roast dinner is, and its usually three or four perfectly vegan items before we get to the meat.

Michael's book reflects how to show care and respect to animals through what we eat, wear and use. It also brilliantly showcases how to recreate the comfort food we all enjoy eating so much. The best vegan food I eat isn't salads, green shakes and lentil bakes, it's flavour-packed burgers, great curries, amazing burritos and fabulous bakes. Just like the recipes you will find in this excellent book.

INTRODUCTION

When I first thought about going vegan, I felt a little peculiar discussing it with my male friends at the pub. They'd say things like 'You'll have no energy!', 'Where will you get your protein from?' and 'Won't you miss meat and cheese?' It was as if they saw meat as a macho, fundamental part of being a man, and I was thinking of removing that from my life. Why? What a ridiculous thing to do!

I've been engaged in a few conversations about veganism that, perhaps when veganism was more obscure than it is now, might easily have taken a nasty turn into mockery and humiliation. Fortunately, successful sportsmen such as heavyweight boxer David Haye, MMA fighter Nate Diaz and champion strongman Patrick Baboumian are demonstrating on the world's stage that veganism doesn't equate to weakness. As veganism becomes normalised and supermarkets' vegan sections grow bigger than ever, the conversation turns more to intrigue than incomprehension.

There are more than 500,000 vegans in the UK, the majority of whom are female. Why? Perhaps because females are stereotypically more sensitive? Or maybe it's that men view vegetarianism and veganism as unmanly and demasculinising. Or are men simply worried about their mates making fun of them? Whatever the cause, the idea that eating a once-conscious being and indirectly contributing to climate change, all the while damaging your own health, is 'part of being a man' is a stereotype that I, as a male, want to firmly reject.

My own transition to a vegan diet started at the beginning of 2016. We'd recently got a dog and, as he quickly became my best pal, I started to question the inconsistency: how can I love him so much but eat other, often equally intelligent and sentient, animals at the same time?

I didn't know much about vegetarianism, let alone veganism. My vegetarian friends were mostly female, and had all been vegetarian since they were tiny – a transition I couldn't relate to. I knew one, maybe two, vegans.

Cruelty to animals was what hooked me into the debate, but I also stumbled upon other information about the impact of animal agriculture on the environment. I (reluctantly!) watched *Cowspiracy*, which, somewhat contrary to my expectations, was an illuminating investigation into the profound effect of animal agriculture on climate change, rather than just a sensationalist and graphic tour of a slaughterhouse. I had continued to eat fish after giving up meat, but I quickly went from pescetarianism to vegetarianism, and then to a

phase I call 'vegan-before-dinner'. I found it far easier to have a vegan breakfast and lunch than the evening meal, which might be cooked by a friend or family member, or even enjoyed at a restaurant. It worked well, until I looked at my dinner and found I was overcompensating for my lack of animal products all day. So, I went 'vegan-until-just-after-dinner'. This quickly ended up being a cheese-binge before bed. Finally, and as I learned more and more about dairy farming, I was able to kick the cheese too – certain mainstream supermarkets' decisions to stock vegan cheese played a big role in this.

To my surprise – particularly as we live in an age in which men's attitude to mental health ('bottle it up', 'don't talk about it', 'get over it') is becoming a huge concern – going vegan had a completely unexpected, and empowering, effect on my mental health. I felt liberated. I had this strange mental clarity in those everyday pauses in activity. I woke up in the morning, believing I was helping myself, and the world, literally by not doing something. When else does inaction result in such good? Around this time I started a blog about the dishes I was experimenting with, and Discover Delicious developed into a place where I shared my excitement about cooking and eating great vegan food.

I do concede that I already knew how to cook, and had a stable and supportive, even interested, home environment. I understand the change may be harder for others to achieve with no time on their hands, no culinary knowledge or a resistant family.

ABOUT THIS BOOK

I hope that my book will provide you with information and guidance that will address any concerns you may have, in addition to an abundance of delicious, tempting, intriguing recipes that won't leave you hungry half an hour later, and more than satisfy your nutritional needs. There are loads of classic recipes, for those of you concerned about missing your favourite meals: full English breakfast, 'chicken' and mushroom pie, lasagne, pasta bake, Indian and Thai curries, burritos, burgers, ramen and falafel wraps. For the athletes and gym-goers among you, I've included a few 'power' recipes that focus on protein and complex carbohydrates. But the book also teaches you how to think in a vegan mindset: there is a bespoke 'Veganise your favourite dishes' section, recipes for vegan basics such as good vegetable stock and vegan mayo, and a guide on how to eat vegan when you're out and about.

Michael Kitson 2018

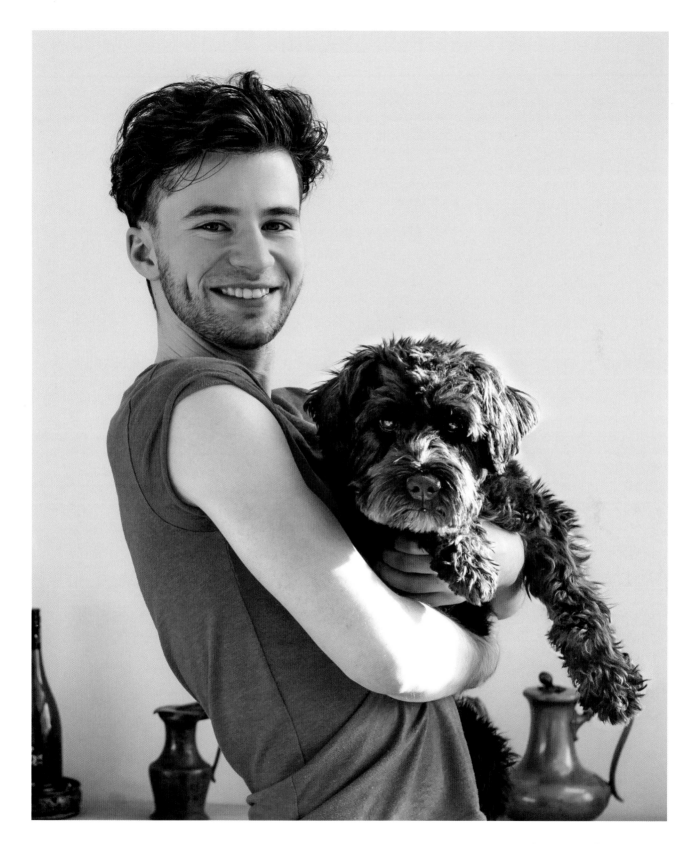

Above *Me and my dog, Max.*

WHY ARE PEOPLE GOING VEGAN?

Broadly speaking, people who refer to themselves as following a 'plant-based' diet are referring to their eating habits only, rather than their lifestyle in general. Plant-based, in a sense, is only one aspect of veganism, which is defined as follows:

'Veganism is a way of living which seeks to exclude, as far as is possible and practicable, all forms of exploitation of, and cruelty to, animals for food, clothing or any other purpose.' (The Vegan Society)

Veganism is not just about food, it addresses various other aspects of our lifestyle, such as clothing – leather from cows, for example – entertainment and animal testing.

Becoming fully vegan can be a process that takes some time, and usually starts with a plant-based diet, which is where this book comes in, offering loads of really tasty food that will inspire newbies and those who have already embraced a vegan lifestyle. But what are the main reasons people are going vegan?

ENVIRONMENT

For some, cruelty to animals is reason enough, but more and more people are also going vegan once they have learned about how farming animals for food affects the environment.

It may come as a surprise to you, but animal agriculture is a major contributor to global warming and climate change. This is because the greenhouse gases created by animal farming, combined with the vast quantities of waste produced by the animals themselves, make up between (estimates vary) 14.5 per cent and a staggering 51 per cent of the world's greenhouse gas emissions.

An inextricably linked concern is the amount of water and land animal agriculture requires. Water is needed to hydrate the animals, but also for growing the huge quantities of grain needed to feed them, and to clean the farm floors. Water is not an unlimited resource, and cleaning the water to make it usable requires lots of energy, creating more greenhouse gases. To give

a more concrete example, 7,700 litres (1,700 gallons) of water will be used in the raising of cattle to produce just 500g (1¼lb) of beef. The production of 500g (1¼lb) of potatoes requires just 144 litres (32 gallons) of water.

The amount of land required to raise animals for food is huge, principally because they consume so much grain. In fact, of all the Amazon rainforest that has been burned or otherwise cleared away, 90 per cent is used to grow grain to feed to farmed animals. It is important to consider the extremely inefficient ratio of grain that farmed animals consume to edible food produced. This grain would be much more efficiently used if it were fed directly to people – for example, sent to a country at high risk of drought and food shortages – rather than to feed 'our' food.

So now you know why meat is so destructive to the environment, what's the situation with fish? The picture ain't much prettier. Catching fish brings its own set of problems: widely used methods such as trawling, which is unregulated in certain parts of the world, lead to a huge amount of bycatch, i.e. catching creatures that were never needed, and have no commercial value, in the first place. Whales, dolphins, turtles and other rare species all fall victim. In addition, these fishing methods destroy coral reefs and wreak havoc on marine ecosystems. And that's not to mention the huge demand for seafood, which has led to overfishing and species extinction.

A little under half of all fish consumed worldwide comes from enclosures known as aquafarms. The density of fish packed into these farms results in quick-spreading diseases and parasites, which farmers seek to address with the overuse of antibiotics, vaccines and pesticides. Some farmed fish are carnivorous, such as salmon, and so are fed wild fish, which

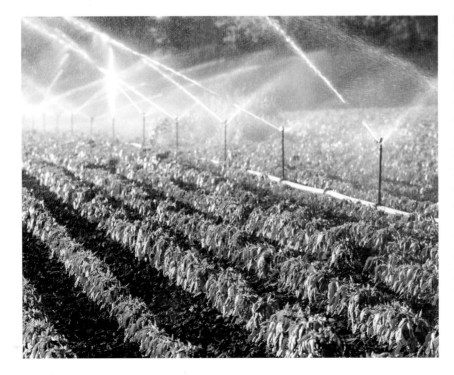

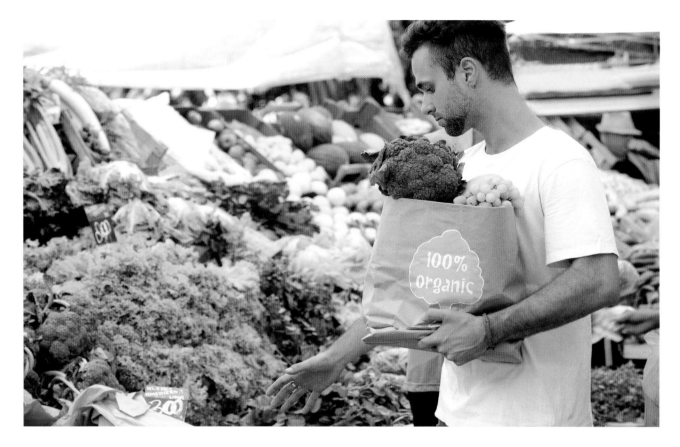

undermines the wild marine food chain and results in an inefficient ratio of food in to food out. Waste from aquafarms (faeces, dead fish and chemicals) pollutes surrounding natural ecosystems when it is flushed from the farm.

HEALTH

As veganism becomes more mainstream, the health benefits of a plant-based diet are reaching a much wider audience. Common health reasons cited for people changing to a plant-based diet include wanting to lose weight, concern over their heart health, research suggesting a link between animal products and cancer, and a lack of energy.

FINANCES

There is a bit of a misconception among some people that eating a healthy vegan diet is going to cost a fortune. This simply isn't the case. Fresh meat, poultry and seafood are increasingly expensive, so cutting out these and a great many processed non-vegan foods immediately

reduces the weekly grocery bill by a not-inconsiderable amount. Vegetables and fruits, especially seasonal, locally produced ones, can be extremely good value for money, while staples such as grains, pulses and even more 'exotic' ingredients such as chia seeds and quinoa are cheaper weight for weight than many animal products.

CONVENIENCE

Being vegan forces you to seek out more independent food stores, local suppliers and restaurants, which is good for the finances of your local community, too. That said, a great many major supermarkets now stock vegan ranges, which are growing at an incredible rate, so with economies of scale kicking in, vegan products are not only more widely and readily available, but are also becoming relatively less expensive than they once were.

Being a more thoughtful shopper, kitchen savvy and batch cooking to take advantage of gluts and bargains will also

help your budget, and sees off the other common misconception: that being a vegan involves a huge amount of time and effort, something that just isn't true.

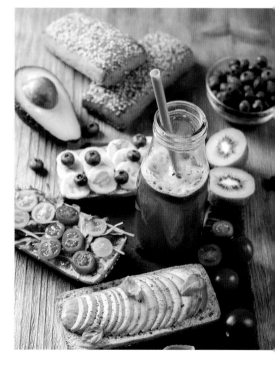

WELL-BEING AND NUTRITION

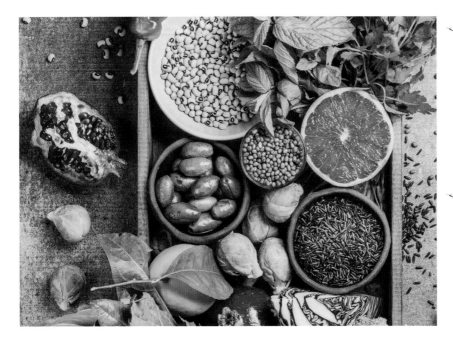

Amid a lot of conflicting arguments and advice, there is some evidence that there could be a link between particular animal products and certain diseases. Processed meat, for example, has been categorised as a potential cause of some cancers by the World Health Organization and there is a less strong, but still positive, indication that some red meat may be carcinogenic. However, since this is primarily a cookbook, rather than going through the often-controversial and ever-changing research and evidence into the risks of eating animal products, I want instead to set out some of the potential health advantages of having a plant-based diet and answer some of the most common questions.

Q *Is a vegan diet healthier than a non-vegan one?*

A While there's no sure-fire way to guarantee you will be healthier on a vegan diet, it is certainly possible. Some of the many benefits include:
- Vegans generally have a much lower risk of type-2 diabetes.

- On average, vegans have lower non-HDL cholesterol levels, blood pressure, BMI and body fat.
- Eliminating meat, dairy and eggs from your diet is likely to significantly reduce your saturated fat intake (though you will need to ensure you consume sufficient fats that are essential for health from other food sources).
- Removing animal products and making space for more plant-based wholefoods significantly increases dietary fibre intake. On average, most people only get about half their daily Reference Intake of fibre.

Q *Can I still be active, play sports and build muscle?*

A Absolutely, for most people and in most instances. See pages 20–1 for a detailed look at exercise, sports and building muscle on a vegan diet.

Q *Is a vegan diet suitable for all the family?*

A Yes, provided you follow the guidelines and maintain a well-planned, well-balanced diet and are prepared to act as the nutritional gatekeeper for your children at school and out and about, as well as at home.

Q *Can I get all the nutrients I need from a vegan diet?*

A Usually, yes – if you include some fortified foods such as plant-based milks. However, if you have a specific medical condition you must always seek and follow your doctor's or dietitian's advice. It is also advisable to seek their advice before considering any major nutritional change to your diet, even if you don't have an underlying condition.

VEGAN NUTRIENT SOURCES
These are the nutrients that are hardest to include or meet the daily Reference Intake for while following a vegan diet, together with a list of good sources:
- **Calcium** – the best plant-based sources are kale, pak choi (bok choy), okra, spring greens, dried figs, chia seeds, almonds, tofu (make sure it has been calcium-set by checking that calcium sulphate is listed in the ingredients) and plant-based milks (some of these are not fortified with calcium – just check for calcium in the ingredients list).
- **Iodine** – this is only naturally present in soil and seawater. It is difficult to ensure a regular, reliable intake of iodine in any diet, especially in the UK, where table salt isn't routinely iodised. The iodine content of fruit and vegetables varies with the amount of iodine present in the soil in which they are grown, which depends on how close to the sea it is. However, it is usually quite low. Seaweed's iodine content is generally very high, but if you buy a type – such as flaked

dulse – that you use in place of, and in the same quantity as, salt, then it's unlikely that you will overdose. Alternatively, you may decide to take it in supplement form.

• **Iron** – beans and lentils, fortified breakfast cereals, dried fruit, dark leafy greens, quinoa and pumpkin seeds are all good sources. Eating foods and drinks high in vitamin C at the same time as eating an iron source improves absorption. See page 21 for more detailed information on iron.

• **Omega-3s – Short answer:** you can get enough of one of the three essential omega-3 fatty acids, Alpha-linolenic Acid (ALA), from walnuts, ground flaxseeds/linseeds, hemp seeds and chia seeds, which can then be turned into the other two fatty acids by your body. However, you need to make sure your omega-6 to omega-3 ratio is low for this to happen, which is difficult, so it may be advisable to take a supplement for the Eicosapentaenoic Acid (EPA) and Docosahexaenoic Acid (DHA) omega-3 fatty acids. Make sure the supplement is vegan!

– **Long answer:** omega-3s are a group of essential – i.e. not made by the body – fatty acids, the most important being: ALA, EPA and DHA. ALA, which can be obtained by eating walnuts, ground flaxseeds/linseeds, hemp seeds and chia seeds, can be turned into EPA by the body. This acid, EPA, can be converted into DHA. It is not easy to get enough DHA on a vegan diet because DHA is almost exclusively found in oily fish. Limiting intake of the omega-6 fatty acid Linoleic Acid (LA), which competes for the enzyme that converts ALA to EPA and then to DHA, is one option for increasing DHA intake on a vegan diet. Most people, vegan or otherwise, have too high a ratio of omega-6 to omega-3 fatty acids, because cheap, widespread oils such as sunflower, corn and soybean oil are so high in omega-6 LA. Vegans tend to have a particularly high omega-6 to omega-3 ratio because nuts, seeds and grains (apart from walnuts, flaxseeds/linseeds, hemp seeds and chia seeds) are higher in omega-6 fats than omega-3s. Cooking with lower-omega-6 oils such as olive, avocado, groundnut (peanut) and rapeseed (canola) is advisable from an omega-3 point of view – in the UK, generic 'vegetable oil' is often made up of mostly rapeseed oil, just check the ingredients on the bottle. Supplementation is an option if you are concerned. You could buy just a DHA, or DHA and EPA supplement, if you are already getting enough ALA from your diet. The latter is easy and quite inexpensive (especially if you grind your own) to do by adding, for example, one heaped dessertspoonful of ground flaxseeds/linseeds to your breakfast cereal. Just make sure the supplement is derived from algae rather than fish oil.

• **Protein** – concentrated plant-based sources are nuts and seeds, seitan, tempeh, tofu, soya mince, (vegan) Quorn and other meat replacements. Other good sources are legumes such as beans, peas, lentils and peanuts; and grains, for example, quinoa and oats. For a more detailed look at protein, see pages 20–1.

• **Selenium** – the content of plant-based sources varies, like iodine, with the soil in which they are grown. Brazil nuts are, on average, the most concentrated source of selenium (including animal products), and you only need one or two per day (they are toxic if eaten in large quantities). However, if these are not to your liking, a supplement is recommended.

• **Vitamin A** – the best foods for vitamin A are pumpkins and squashes, carrots and sweet potatoes, kale and spinach. In addition to eating these foods cooked or raw, some can be juiced raw to provide a real hit.

• **Vitamin B12** –the best sources of B12 for people following a plant-based diet are fortified plant milks or margarine spreads (most are fortified, but check the ingredients to be sure). However, it is highly advisable that vegans take a B12 supplement, to be absolutely certain they get enough.

• **Vitamin D** – we make this hormone ourselves (yes, vitamin D is a hormone!) when our skin is exposed to sunlight. However, in some places and at certain times of the year, light levels are insufficient. The best and easiest plant-based sources are foods fortified with vitamin D such as plant-based milks, but everyone, not just vegans, is advised by the NHS to consider a vitamin D supplement during autumn and winter, when getting it from sunlight and/or food can be difficult. Vitamins D2 and D3 are both eventually turned into vitamin D by the body. If given the choice, choose D3 as a supplement.

• **Vitamin K** – vitamin K1 is found in green vegetables, such as cabbage, spinach, kale, spring greens, broccoli, Brussels sprouts and kiwis. Vitamin K2 can be synthesised by our bodies from K1.

• **Zinc** – good sources include beans, lentils, tofu, chickpeas, cashew nuts, walnuts, chia seeds, hemp seeds, pumpkin seeds and ground flaxseeds/linseeds, wholemeal (whole-wheat) bread and quinoa.

DIETARY SUPPLEMENTS

The easiest solution if you are concerned you are not getting enough of certain nutrients is to take a supplement that has been specifically developed for vegans. If the one you choose doesn't include omega-3 fatty acids, you may want to buy a separate omega-3 supplement that contains DHA, or EPA and DHA – make sure it is derived from algae and not fish.

INGREDIENTS TO AVOID AND WHY

Some non-vegan foods – such as eggs, fish and lactose, which are very commonly used in processed foods and in restaurants – are also common allergens, which means that they are emphasised in bold, italics or underlined on the back of food packaging and may be listed in menus, making it easier to spot them. It goes without saying, though, that this only applies to allergens rather than non-vegan foods, so you do need to pay attention to what is in food so you can avoid ones that aren't suitable for vegans. These are listed below, with information on why vegans avoid them.

It is important to preface the following information with the statement, which most vegans will agree with (but not all), that being a vegan is not always black and white. If you eat a cookie that contains 0.001 grams of monoglycerides that may possibly be animal-derived, does that mean you are not vegan? No. If you order an alcohol drink without checking online whether or not it has been filtered with animal products, does that mean

you're no longer vegan? No. Or how about if you go to your grandma's house and eat the cake she has kindly made you, even though it contains eggs, are you then not a vegan? Again, no. It is essential to think about why you lead, or are increasingly trying to lead, a vegan lifestyle. Absolutism and being overly pedantic are unnecessary and in the end will just put you (and other people) off. Most vegans will agree it is better for the world, the animals and yourself to have an occasional accidental, or even purposeful, slip-up, than to do nothing at all.

MEAT, POULTRY, FISH, SHELLFISH, DAIRY AND EGGS

These are, of course, the primary foods to avoid when following a vegan diet and it goes without saying (hopefully) that they shouldn't be eaten in any form whatsoever. Some are more obvious and easily avoided than others; eggs and dairy appear in so many unexpected foods, so you really do need to be vigilant and

check packaging. Or just make your own, rather than relying on packaged food (which is why you bought this book, right?).

HONEY

A lot of people are surprised that honey isn't vegan. You might think 'but bees make honey anyway, why can't we take some for ourselves?'. Unfortunately, it's not as simple as that. Beekeepers replace the honey in hives with a nutritionally inadequate sugar substitute, which results in malnourished, unhealthy bees. This is exacerbated by bees exhausting themselves, overworking to replace the missing honey.

Malnourishment and overwork, combined with selective breeding to up productivity (which depletes the gene pool), all increase bees' susceptibility to disease. This can have knock-on effects as disease then spreads to other pollinators on which ecosystems and animals rely.

Fortunately, honey is one of the easiest foods to replace. Maple, agave and golden (light corn) syrup (as well as dark muscovado and other sugars) are delicious alternatives that work well in baking and as a spread or sweetener.

GELATINE

Made from boiled bones, gelatine crops up in many processed foods, from sweets (candies) and chewing gum to mousses, cheesecakes, jellies and all manner of other baked and factory-made foods. Vegan versions made with agar agar are increasingly available, but do check packaging really carefully.

ALCOHOLIC BEVERAGES

Some producers of wine, beer and spirits choose to use animal products to clarify their beverages. Common filtering agents

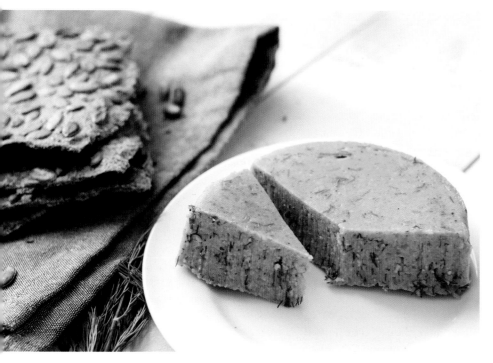

Left *Nut cheeses, like this cashew cheese with chives, are increasingly available.*

include isinglass (a substance derived from dried swim bladders of fish), sea shells, gelatine and egg whites.

Fortunately, there is also a rapidly increasing number of producers who don't use these agents, so you can still enjoy thousands of beers, wines, ciders and spirits. It is worth noting, though, that these producers sometimes miss a trick and don't label their products as 'suitable for vegans', even if they are. To help clarify the matter, www.barnivore.com is an excellent website that lists whether or not thousands of alcoholic beverages are vegan – and you can always contact the producer of a drink to which you are particularly partial to check, too.

Here is a general rules of thumb (but do check, as things change and differ around the world):

- Most mega-corp beer, whether it's in a bottle, can or from a keg, is vegan. Such big name beers include Carlsberg, Heineken, Stella Artois, Budweiser, etc.
- Ale from a cask (note: casks are different from kegs) is generally produced using isinglass. A notable exception is Samuel Smith's cask ales (apart from their Brewery Bitter).
- Modern craft beer and ale producers frequently offer vegan beverages. Brewdog, Marble and Moor are popular craft brewers that don't use any animal products.
- There are beer purity laws in Germany and Belgium so, generally speaking, beers brewed there won't contain animal products.
- Wines are quite hit-and-miss. Some of the Co-op, Sainsbury's, Asda, Waitrose and Tesco own-brand wines are vegan, and the Co-op and Sainsbury's are particularly good at labelling whether or not their wines are vegan friendly.
- Popular ciders such as Kopparberg, Strongbow and Rekorderlig unfortunately include gelatine in their

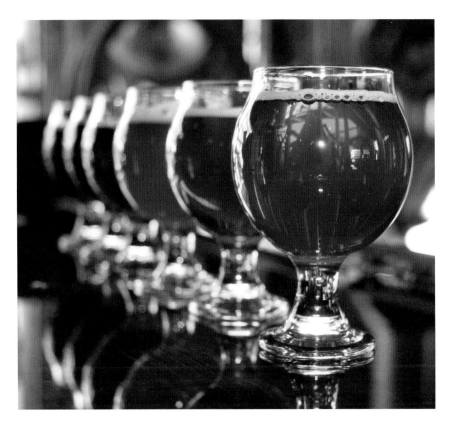

manufacturing (so they're not even suitable for vegetarians). However, Bulmers, Aspall and pear-flavoured Magners and Strongbow are suitable for vegans.
- Most spirits are suitable for vegans.

PALM OIL

Palm oil, on the face of it, is a vegan substance: an edible oil extracted from the fruit of a tree called the African oil palm. What makes the oil a global issue, and why some vegans avoid it, is the method used to retrieve the palm fruits. The oil is in such high demand that massive areas of the Amazon rainforest have been burned or otherwise cleared away to make room for oil palm trees, a process that not only leads to soil erosion and pollutes waterways but also destroys animal habitats and often leads to their deaths. This exacerbates the plights of already endangered species, such as, to name but a few, orangutans, rhinos, elephants and tigers.

What's more, the deliberate burning of the rainforest releases CO_2, which

pollutes local villages and contributes to global warming. Lastly, illegal production of palm oil has been known to result in children being used as labourers and can involve other human rights abuses.

Fortunately, there are now products that use sustainably sourced palm oil. Sometimes this is not explicitly stated, though, so you could avoid that product to be safe or, if you're really interested, have a look at the manufacturer's palm oil policy. For example, Unilever, which makes Stork (block margarine used for baking), launched a Sustainable Palm Oil Sourcing Policy in 2016, but this responsible sourcing information is not stated on the packaging.

MILK-DERIVED PRODUCTS

Whey (powder, protein or other forms), casein and lactoglobulin are ingredients sometimes used in processed foods. Food packaging nearly always highlights these ingredients (e.g. in bold) or have the words '(from milk)' written next to them. They should be avoided.

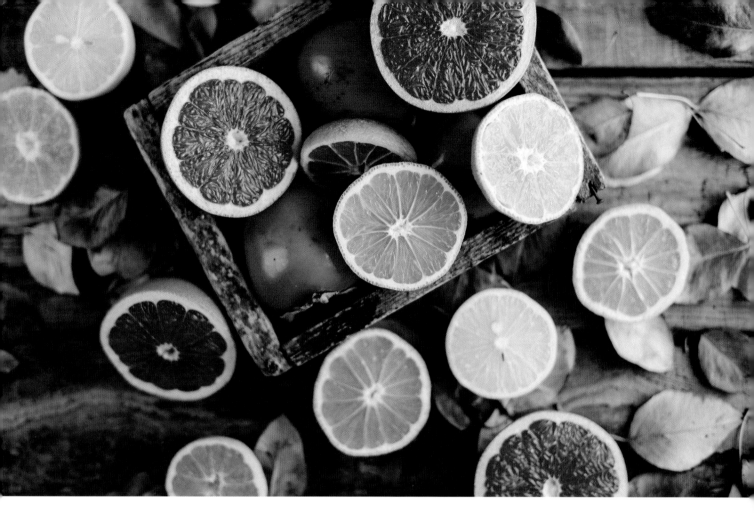

PASTES, SAUCES AND CONDIMENTS

Some pastes and sauces, particularly from South East Asian countries, e.g. Thai green curry paste, contain fish sauce or shrimp paste. Closer to home, watch out for Worcestershire Sauce, which contains anchovies. Happily, there are Thai curry pastes and other Asian staples that don't contain these fishy ingredients – just be sure to read the labels carefully – and Henderson's Relish, which is similar to Worcestershire Sauce but is vegan-friendly. You can also use alternatives to add an umami hit, such as seaweed, mushrooms and mushroom ketchup.

WAXED FRUIT AND VEGETABLES

Some fresh produce, especially citrus fruits and apples, are often coated in wax that is made from shellac (derived from the lac bug) or beeswax, which is a no-no, or petroleum or palm oil, which still isn't great, albeit technically suitable for vegans. Since it is very hard to know what type of wax has been used, it's best to simply avoid waxed produce.

L-CYSTEINE

Derived from poultry feathers, this amino acid is sometimes added to breads, bagels and other baked foods to serve as a softening agent. Look out for it in ingredients lists.

E-NUMBERS

E-numbers are safety classification codes for food additives. Certain E-numbers stand for ingredients that are always derived from animals, and there there are a few contentious ones that can be derived from either animals or plants. Listed below are the numbers that are always animal-derived and should be avoided if possible.

- **E120** – carminic acid is a red dye and food colouring made from cochineal insects. It is commonly found in shockingly red or pink alcohol beverages (not the only reason to stay away from those). Maraschino cherries also use the stuff. If a food seems more pink than it otherwise might, it may well contain E120.
- **E542** – edible bone phosphate made from cattle or pig bones. Used in cosmetics and toothpaste and (very rarely) as an anti-caking agent in some ground substances such as dried milk (which you no longer need to worry about!), salt and baking powder.
- **E901** – beeswax. Frequently used in candles, cosmetics, sometimes confectionery and to coat fruit.
- **E904** – shellac, a resin secreted by the lac insect. Although it's a secretion, retrieval methods mean around 25 per cent of this substance is made up of crushed insects. It can be used to polish furniture, in instruments, for sweets (candies), to coat pills and your finger nails, and even (rarely) apples. Obviously, non-food items such as furniture do not have ingredients labels. If you are very keen to avoid it, you'll have to do some prior research on your purchase.

WHAT NOT TO WEAR, USE OR BUY

If you're reading this book because you want to change your diet in order to better your health, that's great, a really positive thing to do, and can only be encouraged. However, it would also be more appropriately labelled as wanting to follow a plant-based diet, rather than lead a vegan lifestyle.

As the definition on page 10 states, veganism is not a diet but an ethical mind set and way of living that seeks to reduce the suffering of animals as far as is possible and practicable. This extends to the clothes you wear, cosmetics you use and activities you pursue.

CLOTHING AND MATERIALS
Aside from altering your diet, the most common change people make in order to reduce animal suffering is to abstain from wearing clothes made from animal skins or coats. There are three reasons, which can be broadly extended to most animal by-product industries, why using animal by-products is unethical:

1. cruel practices are often employed to speed up production;
2. the animal itself needs the product and has to die or suffer in order for us to use it instead;
3. continuing to buy these goods perpetuates the demand for the farming, and slaughter, of animals.

The material with the most obvious ethical issues is leather, which is made from a variety of animal hides (not just cow – pig, goat and sheep are also used). While some may regard the animal hide as a by-product of the meat industry, which would otherwise go to waste, this is not the case. Roughly 10 per cent of the animal's value at the abattoir lies with its skin, so buying leather is directly funding the meat industry. What's more, leather most commonly comes from developing countries such as China and India, where animal welfare laws are often largely either non-existent or unenforced.

Wool, silk, fur, suede and cashmere, as well as items made from down, all involve aspects of cruelty and exploitation, too, and their purchase perpetuates their industries.

It can be overwhelming to see how far animal materials pervade our lifestyles and habits. Briefcases, wallets, pillows, duvets, car seats, sofas, scarves and rugs can all be made from animal skins or coats or feathers, as well as all the clothes, shoes and boots. Fortunately, it's easier than ever to avoid these materials. Synthetic leather is widely available, cheaper and can even be stronger than real leather. In fact, it is easy to buy practical and fashionable clothing from ordinary clothes stores or websites, as

a great many are made from synthetic materials, such as acrylic or polyester. Non-down bedding is also readily available, much cheaper and often hypoallergenic.

There are lots of vegan websites and forums now that share information on where to buy clothes made without animal materials.

COSMETICS AND TOILETRIES
Encouragingly, testing on animals for cosmetic products is banned in the European Union (although some companies still test on animals overseas for markets abroad). However, since Britain voted to leave the EU, the future laws will be up to the British government to decide. At the time of publication, testing on animals for cosmetics is still banned in Britain.

The safest bet, wherever you are in the world, is simply to look on the product's packaging for a leaping bunny logo, the emblem of Cruelty-Free International, to ensure your cosmetics and toiletries are cruelty free. There are some other schemes around the world, too, so always check to be sure.

Online sources will again help on finding cosmetics and toiletries that have not been tested on animals, and many top brands now offer their own ranges of vegan products.

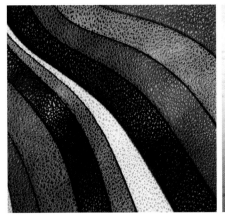
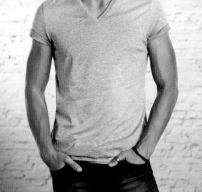
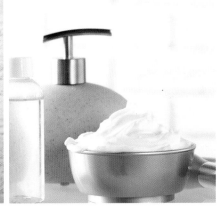

VEGANISM ON THE GO

It's all very well following a vegan lifestyle when you are in charge of your own food, but it can be a bit of a minefield when you are out and about, especially if you have other people's tastes and preferences to contend with. Fortunately, there are many ways to make life easier for yourself, and as veganism grows, it is only going to get better. The following recommendations are correct at the time of publication, but be wary as they are subject to change as brands alter recipes and restaurants change their menus.

SNACKS AND TAKEAWAY FOOD

When at work, on an outing or otherwise on the go, most people tend to buy food that is nearby and convenient. Of course if you're willing to plan ahead you can make your own – but sometimes you just have to buy food on the hoof. On the face of it, you may think you'll be at the whim of high street chains and supermarkets, but there's been a recent explosion in the number of independent vegan cafes, delis and restaurants in towns and cities, so with a little research it's likely you'll be able to find somewhere that sells great, tasty, nutritious takeaway vegan food that doesn't require you to go too far afield. Or you can order it to your desk.

Even major international chains are starting to up their vegan game and provide more choice, but if all else fails then there's always supermarkets, which are also increasing their vegan ranges, even in their convenience stores. What's more, for those times when you are tired and stressed and don't have time to seek out or make healthier choices, there have always been lots of 'accidentally vegan' items for sale that will satisfy a craving for instant gratification. These include:

- Instant noodles – these are a convenient option for work, and, bizarrely, sometimes the 'meaty' ones, are vegan! Do, however, check the

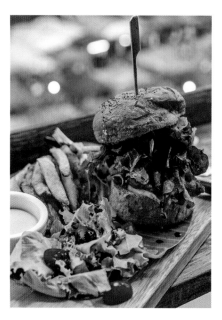

ingredients list carefully for E-numbers and hidden animal products, and bear in mind the salt content. Some are healthier than others, so shop around and perhaps don't rely on them on a daily basis.
- Crisps (US potato chips) – you can satisfy your savoury, salty cravings with many different crisps – even 'bacon'-flavoured ones tend to use flavouring and are suitable for vegans.
- Crackers – Ritz or cream crackers can be spread with supermarket guacamole, hummus or even Lotus Biscuit Spread for a cheeky snack at your desk.
- Protein bars – quite a few of the major brands are vegan and these are very widely available. Although they may seem quite expensive, they are more nutritious than most of the above, and can be eaten on the go or shoved in a bag to fend off an attack of the munchies on the way home.
- Naughty but nice sweet treats – sometimes we all want/need a sugar hit to keep us going, which is where store-bought sweets (candies), cookies and cakes can come to the

rescue. Although many do contain animal products, quite a few are vegan friendly, including Skittles, some Haribo, Oreos, ginger nuts (gingersnaps), fig rolls, Rich Tea, digestive and bourbon biscuits, and some of the Mr Kipling range. And many, many more besides.

DINING OUT

Following a vegan diet can make going to a restaurant tricky, especially when you want to go out with non-vegan friends and family. Twenty or even 10 years ago, the situation might have been very disheartening, but happily the outlook now is much more encouraging and in recent years veganism has taken off into mainstream society. Increased demand has led to vegan options appearing in high street restaurant chains and sparked the creation of bespoke vegan restaurants and pop-ups. What's more, the trend for vegan 'junk food' has led to veganism losing its halo; it is no longer regarded as a diet of deprivation and worthiness. You will now find stores and stalls selling anything from vegan döner kebabs to greasy fried 'chicken'.

If you're eating out with non-vegan friends, many high street chain restaurants now offer vegan dishes – sometimes even whole vegan menus! – including (but not limited to): Wagamama, Zizzi, Wetherspoons, Pizza Express, Las Iguanas and All Bar One. And these are just a few of the chains in the UK – elsewhere, these and others will offer up all sorts of different options, so get online and see what's available.

If your group chooses an independent, local restaurant over a chain, don't despair! It's often relatively painless. For example, Middle Eastern restaurants often have 'accidentally vegan' items such as falafel and hummus, Indian restaurants will always have a variety of vegetarian options, some of which may be vegan, and if the pizza restaurant doesn't have vegan cheese in stock, just skip the cheese and pile on some olive-oily roasted veggies. Another option, perhaps for the proactive and less shy, is just to ask the chef to make your dish vegan. They are often up to the task, and can perhaps tweak a dish just by removing a known animal product from the vegetarian option.

If, however, your friends want to go to a fast food chain that is generally meat heavy, such as McDonald's, Subway or Burger King, you won't have to go hungry. The following information should help you out, though of course the menu does change and could also vary depending on where in the world you are, so do check:

- **McDonald's** – the hash browns and fries are vegan, as is the Vegetable Deluxe without 'sandwich sauce'.
- **Subway** – the Veggie Delite is vegan, as long as you don't add cheese and avoid the 9-grain Honey Oat bread, Italian Herbs & Cheese and the Flatbread. The BBQ, Sweet Onion and Sweet Chilli sauces are all vegan.
- **KFC** – fries (skin-on or off), baked beans and the corn cob are vegan.
- **Nando's** – for a starter, the Houmus, Mixed Olives and PERI-PERI nuts are all vegan. Go for the Supergreen or Sweet Potato & Butternut in a burger, pitta or wrap as a main – just ask for no mayo. Garlic bread, ordinary or PERI-salted chips (fries) and Chargrilled Veg both work as a side. The Mango Sorbet for dessert is vegan.
- **Pizza Hut** – all UK Pizza Hut restaurants offer vegan cheese. Just make sure you pick the Pan, All American Thin or Flatbread base. Oh, and their bacon bits are vegan!
- **Domino's** – unfortunately their bases contain a milk-derived ingredient. Their potato wedges are the only vegan option.
- **Burger King** – unfortunately only their fries are vegan-friendly. And their ketchup.

Lastly, it's a good idea to download the app Happy Cow, which you can use to find nearby restaurants and cafes that have vegan options. It covers the UK, USA and other areas of the world.

OUTINGS

I know it sounds sort of killjoy-esque, but vegans – like lots of non-vegans – generally don't support or visit zoos or aquariums. Both provide fractional space and freedom to the animals compared with what they would have in the wild. Some argue that zoos help with animal conservation, and while this may be true, these attractions are businesses, and so mostly have 'popular' animals that people want to see, such as lions, gorillas and dolphins. If your children really want to get up close to some animals, you could take them to see happy, rescued animals at an sanctuary instead of a zoo.

Horse and greyhound racing also go against vegan principles as they exploit animals for entertainment and can involve cruel practices behind the scenes.

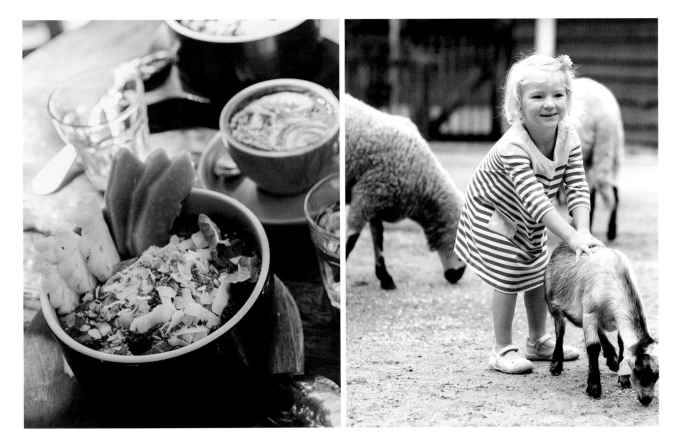

EXERCISE AND BUILDING MUSCLE

If you enjoy sport and exercise, you might be concerned about whether you can continue with your activities when you switch to a plant-based diet.

The perception that veganism equates to weakness and inadequate protein is being proven untrue. Quite the reverse, in fact; vegan athletes can and do match and even surpass the performance of their non-vegan competitors. Below are responses to some of the most commonly asked questions:

Q *Is it possible to exercise, play sport and thrive on a vegan diet?*

A Yes, for most people, most of the time. As demonstrated by many famous vegan athletes, you can thrive on a vegan diet whether you are anything from a bodybuilder to an endurance runner. These successful sportsmen, from a variety of sports, all follow a plant-based diet:

- David Haye, heavyweight boxer
- Patrik Baboumian, holds title 'Strongest Man in Germany'
- David Carter, NFL player
- Scott Jurek, ultramarathon champion
- Nate Diaz, MMA fighter
- Jermain Defoe, Premier League and England footballer
- Anthony Mullally, Leeds Rhinos rugby league player

Q *Can I get enough protein?*

A The most frequently asked question vegans receive is 'where do you get your protein from?' It becomes especially relevant here, because to build muscle you need between (estimates vary) 1.7 to 2.4 times the Reference Intake (RI) of protein. This means that

Right Soy products, like tempeh and tofu, are good sources of protein.

if you want to increase muscle, you should be aiming for 1.3 to 1.8 grams of protein per kilogram of bodyweight, since the normal RI for maintenance of bodyweight is 0.75 grams of protein per kg bodyweight.

It is indeed possible to get enough protein to build muscle on a vegan diet, if you plan your diet and eat the correct foods. The following are excellent sources of protein:

- **Seitan** – up to 30g/1½oz protein per 100g/3¾oz
- **Nuts and seeds** – up to 30g/1½oz protein per 100g/3¾oz
- **Tempeh** – 20g/¾oz protein per 100g/3¾oz
- **Soya mince and other soya meat-replacement products** – 15g/½oz protein per 100g/3¾oz
- **Edamame beans** – 13g/scant ½ oz protein per 100g/3¾oz
- **Tofu** – 12g/scant ½ oz protein per 100g/3¾oz

Other wholefood sources:
- **Quinoa** – 13g/scant ½ oz protein per 100g/3¾oz
- **Lentils** – 9g/¼oz protein per 100g/3¾oz
- **Black beans and chickpeas** – 8g/¼oz protein per 100g/3¾oz

If your diet is centred around foods such as these, and you eat enough calories, then you'll have no problem getting sufficient protein. However, if you are still unconvinced, there are plant-based protein powders available.

Bodybuilders and weightlifters may have to focus more on eating enough calories because they are used to eating meat, which is often calorifically dense. A diet centred around complex carbohydrates such as brown rice, sweet potatoes and beans, with some nuts and seeds (high in healthy fats and protein and so very calorifically dense), should provide enough calories.

Q *But are they 'complete' proteins?*

A A common misconception is that you can't get 'complete' proteins from plant-based sources – that is,

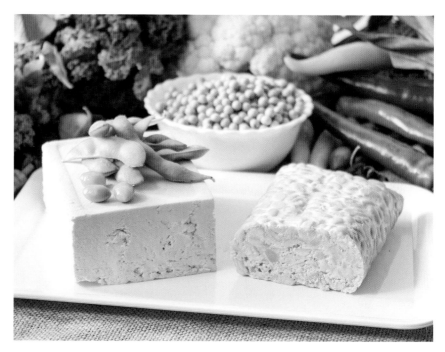

protein that contains all nine essential amino acids. Fortunately, there is no truth to this. There are two strategies. One is to include pumpkin seeds, buckwheat, quinoa, hemp seeds or soya products such as edamame beans, tofu and tempeh in your diet, which are all complete proteins in and of themselves.

The second, which will sometimes happen without you even thinking about it, is to combine a couple of plant-based foods to make sure you get all nine essential amino acids. This really isn't difficult. Lysine tends to be the limiting essential amino acid in a vegan diet as it is present in low quantities in most plant-based foods, except for legumes. So, as long as you combine legumes (beans, lentils, peas, peanuts) with non-legume plant-based sources of protein such as nuts, oats, brown rice, quinoa and other wholegrains, then you will obtain all nine essential amino acids. These don't have to be eaten at the same time, either; the liver stores the various essential amino acids so you can eat them at different times of the day.

Q *Are there any advantages to eating a vegan diet with regard to sporting endeavours?*

A For some people, yes. Some sportspeople who follow a very carefully planned and controlled vegan diet see a reduction in fatigue and recovery time, which allows them to train more frequently and reach levels of performance previously unattainable. This subsequent increased endurance is what persuades some athletes to make the change.

The potential to increase pace and agility is another tempting benefit for many active people. For example, David Haye and Nate Diaz, boxing and MMA fighters respectively, adopted a plant-based diet because they found the diet increased their speed.

What's more, it's likely that you'll be healthier in general. Broadly speaking, plant-based sources of protein come

in a package with fibre, vitamins and minerals and low amounts of saturated fat and cholesterol. If you fill your diet with these plant-based wholefoods, your cardiovascular health and resistance to disease will probably improve.

There are various micronutrients essential to athletic performance that might be easier to get on a vegan diet that usually involves you eating more vegetables and fruits. These include:

- **Potassium**, vital in the transportation and storage of carbohydrates to fuel muscles, found in avocados, mushrooms, buckwheat, legumes and greens.
- **Vitamin C** to increase iron absorption, found in oranges, mangoes, grapefruit, broccoli and red (bell) peppers.
- **Vitamin A** to protect against oxidative damage from exercise. Vitamin A can be found in pumpkins, squashes, carrots, sweet potatoes, kale and spinach.
- **Magnesium** is hard to get from animal products. It plays an important role in muscle contractions and the metabolic process. Leafy greens, nuts (especially cashews and almonds), seeds, legumes and grains are all rich in magnesium.

Q *What about iron?*

A Iron deficiency can lead to poor energy levels and fatigue, and so is especially important when it comes to working out and exercise. Impact endurance sportspeople, in particular runners, can have issues with their iron levels as a result of a condition called foot strike haemolysis (the repeated action of striking the ground damages red blood cells, meaning they have to be replaced more quickly, which uses up more iron). Most people can normally get enough iron on a vegan diet, though people who do a significant amount of training should seek advice from a dietitian and follow a carefully formulated and personalised eating plan. Legumes

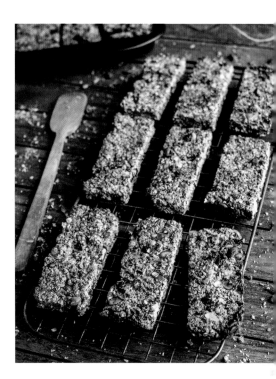

(beans, lentils, peas, peanuts), grains, fortified breakfast cereals, dried fruit and dark leafy greens, quinoa and pumpkin seeds are all good sources. To bolster your intake, and this is important, eat a food that is rich in vitamin C, such as citrus fruits, strawberries, green leafy vegetables (broccoli, kale, collards, Swiss chard, Brussels sprouts), (bell) peppers (yellow, red, and green), and cauliflower, alongside your iron source to significantly improve absorption. Avoid coffee and all teas at meal times as they contain polyphenols that inhibit iron absorption.

PROTEIN-RICH RECIPES

The Protein-packed Porridge on page 41 is an excellent, fuelling start to the day, as is the Date & Banana Smoothie on page 36. For a pre- and post-workout snack, or just an afternoon lift, try out the Power Bars (pictured above) on page 56. Made of oats, chia seeds and almond butter, each bar packs in a pleasing hit of plant-based protein. See Power Bowl I and Power Bowl II on pages 90 and 93 for recipes that combine grains, beans, greens, nuts and seeds for a complex, protein-high and delicious meal.

STORECUPBOARD ESSENTIALS AND USEFUL INGREDIENTS FOR VEGAN COOKING

Listed below are some ingredients frequently used in vegan cooking (besides the obvious and hopefully already familiar fruit, vegetables, pulses, nuts, seeds etc), alongside an explanation of what they are, what they are used for, and why. It may be handy to have some of these stocked in your cupboard.

You will also find certain obscure ingredients listed. I can assure you that these unfamiliar ingredients aren't used just to make your shopping trip that little bit more difficult – I've included them mainly to provide a vegan substitute for the flavour or texture of recipes that are traditionally made with animal products.

FLAXSEED AND CHIA SEEDS

Flaxseed, aka linseeds, are very frequently used in vegan cooking as an egg replacer. Soaked in water, they thicken into a binding gel for use in baking, binding 'meatballs' and other mixtures.

In addition to their binding quality, flaxseed/linseeds are also the most concentrated plant-based source of omega-3 Alpha-linolenic Acid, an added bonus to using them in baked goods (more on this on page 13). Of course, you could just sprinkle the ground seeds on your food for the same benefit, just note that whole flaxseed/linseeds will not have the same effect as ground ones since they are not digested by the body.

Once a pack of ground flaxseed/linseeds is opened it should be stored in the fridge as the omega-3 fats are volatile and will quickly go rancid.

CHIA SEEDS

Chia seeds have the remarkable ability to absorb nine times their own volume in water. They have many similarities with ground flaxseed/linseeds as, soaked in water for 15 minutes, they too thicken into a thick, gloopy gel. The main

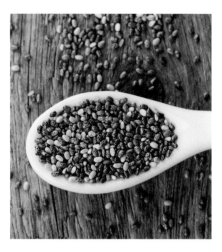

difference between flaxseeds/linseeds and chia seeds is that chia seeds (pictured above) don't have to be ground. Chia seeds are also more expensive.

But which one should you use? Generally speaking, ground flaxseed/linseeds work better as a binder for cakes, cookies and other baked goods, as well as for vegan meatballs and burgers. Chia seeds are better for uncooked recipes, for example in 'chia puddings'.

CORNFLOUR (CORNSTARCH)

Used for centuries as a thickener in mainstream cooking, cornflour is also often used to replicate thick dairy products in vegan recipes. For example, it is used for texture in the Lemon No-bake Cheesecake recipe on page 139.

BUTTER SUBSTITUTES

Vegan butter substitutes can be classified into two groups: spreads and baking block margarine.

- Spreads are used for exactly that: to spread on toast or crackers. They generally consist of various vegetable oils and are solid if kept in the fridge. They claim they can be used for baking and cooking, but they have a high water content, and I would always

recommend baking block margarine instead for that purpose.

- Baking block margarine comes in foil, just like dairy butter, and is often simply (and rather vaguely) referred to as 'baking block'. In American recipes, it is called 'vegan butter'. Frequently, something along the lines of 'best for Biscuits & Pastry' is specified on the front of the packaging. Stork is a well-known brand, but supermarkets often stock an own-brand version. Baking block margarine is the best butter substitute for cakes, cookies and other baked goods where the texture is important. It is used a lot in this book, and is always referred to as 'baking block margarine'.

PLANT-BASED MILKS

These 'milks' can be made from a number of ingredients. The varieties most commonly found in stores come from soya beans, almonds, oats and rice. More obscure milks are available, such as hemp, cashew nut and hazelnut.

Plant-based milks are most frequently made by soaking the bean, nut or grain in water, blending it, and then straining the mixture to leave a smooth white liquid. Sometimes a sweetener is added, which I prefer – perhaps because dairy milk, which I, and most people, grew up on, is actually quite high in sugar (in the form of lactose). Helpfully, many plant-based milks are fortified with some or all of vitamins B2, B12, D, E, as well as calcium. It is highly advisable to buy a fortified plant-milk.

You can make your own plant-based milk, but I personally don't bother. It's a long, laborious, rather boring process and the final product doesn't even taste better. What's more, plant-based milks are now widely available, relatively inexpensive, and are fortified with essential nutrients (unlike a homemade one). Buying them instead is a no-brainer in my book (which this is).

Choosing the right plant-based milk to use can be overwhelming given the huge variety of choices. In my experience, everyone finds their favourite eventually by a process of trial and error. A lot of people don't like the taste of the cheapest option – usually own-brand unsweetened soya milk – but it thickens well, so often works in cooking. For drinking, I've found hazelnut milk, though pricey, is utterly delectable, but that's just my opinion. You should also consider where the milk comes from and how it was produced, and try to go for one whose production hasn't involved land clearance or excessive amounts of water. Almond milk in particular gets a bad rap on this front, but do bear in mind that it is still better for the environment than dairy milk.

What about our old friend, canned coconut milk? Is that a trendy plant-based milk? In essence, it is indeed a plant-based milk and is made in a relatively similar way, but coconut milk is different in that it is much thicker and less diluted than most drinking plant-based milks, is very high in fat,

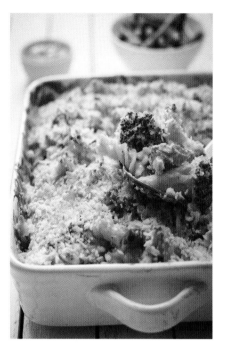

and is intended for cooking. It makes an excellent alternative to dairy cream and is used a lot in this book, particularly in Asian and Indian recipes. Don't confuse it with coconut 'drink', sold in cartons, intended for drinking and as a replacement for dairy milk.

Below left *nut milks*. Below *Almond butter overnight oats (page 37)*.

CASHEW NUTS

I'm not sure how someone discovered this, but if you soak cashew nuts in water, they plump up and can then be blended into a rich, creamy sauce. With the addition of flavourings such as nutritional yeast, onion powder and garlic powder, it can be used to replace thick dairy-based sauces, for instance in the Pasta Bake with Creamy Cashew Sauce (pictured left) on page 107.

Cashew nuts can also be used to make a kind of tzatziki (pictured below), recipe on page 58, cream cheese, sour cream, or fermented cheese. You can make these yourself or purchase them – there are now small artisan companies producing a variety of cashew cheeses. Alternatively, soaked cashew nuts can be used for sweet recipes, again to replace dairy – in vegan cheesecakes or tiramisu.

Recipes normally recommend that you soak the cashew nuts in water overnight or for at least 3 hours. This will produce the best results, but you can get around it by either soaking them in boiling water for just 15 minutes. The result won't be as creamy or smooth, but will still work. A high-powered blender yields the best results; it is difficult to properly blend cashews with a stick blender.

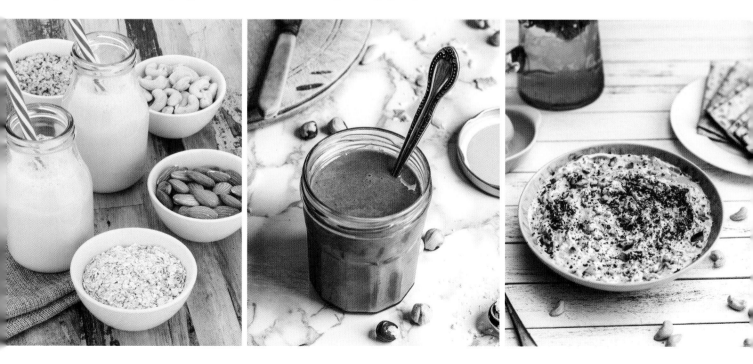

NUTRITIONAL YEAST

This product wins the award for most unappealing food name. Which is unfortunate, because it's an excellent ingredient to have to hand. People sometimes refer to it as 'nooch'.

Nutritional yeast is essentially yeast that has been grown, heated (to deactivate it), and dried. It has a vibrant yellow colour and a surprisingly cheesy flavour, more akin to 'American' cheese, than an artisanal, expensive, aged cheese. It can be sprinkled on to food or, more frequently, used to give sauces a cheesy flavour. A vegan cauliflower cheese sauce will certainly make use of the stuff. Another example is as a substitute for Parmesan in pesto. It is almost always fortified with vitamin B12.

In the UK, the most common brand is Engevita, but other brands are available too. It is also called 'nutritional yeast flakes' or 'savoury yeast flakes'.

ONION GRANULES/POWDER/ DRIED ONIONS

Made from ground, dehydrated onions, this product is mild, with none of the harshness of fresh, raw onion, and has a faintly nutty, cheesy flavour. It is much more commonly found on the spice racks of homes in the USA than in the UK, and is referred to and bought as powder there rather than granules. The granules available in the UK are far better if you grind them to a powder.

Onion powder is often used in commercial rubs and marinades, but I highly recommend buying some as it adds a rounded, savoury, cheesy element to your sauces or dips. .

GARLIC GRANULES/POWDER

This is made using the same technique as onion granules: dehydrating and grinding fresh garlic. It tastes a little garlicky, with only a hint of the powerful bite that fresh garlic possesses. It's commonly used in spice blends and marinades, and often paired with onion granules/powder. If you can find garlic powder, buy that, as it can be incorporated more easily into sauces and dips than granules.

KALA NAMAK (AKA INDIAN BLACK SALT)

A volcanic rock salt harvested in the Himalayas, kala namak is very high in sulphur, which gives it an aroma and taste reminiscent of hard-boiled eggs. It can be used in vegan dishes to replicate the flavour of eggs – it is extremely pungent at first but less so once cooked. When ground, despite the name, it is more of a light mauve colour. In whole crystals it is more of a browny-purple. It's quite hard to find; you'll have to travel to an Asian supermarket or purchase it online. Just don't get it confused with 'black ritual salt', which is inedible and is used for sprinkling around your house to protect it from intruders... no comment.

KOMBU (DRIED KELP)

This seaweed comes in quite large sheets, and is one of the two components in a classic Japanese dashi stock (alongside dried bonito (tuna) flakes). It adds a seaweed-y, umami savouriness to soups, stews and stocks. You can buy it in most Asian supermarkets, at online seaweed stores and, increasingly, in regular supermarkets. If you wash it, you will lose some flavour, so just gently wipe any dirt away – and don't clean off the white powder as it contains the salty flavour and minerals.

Below left *nutritional yeast.* Below *kala namak,* Below right *kombu.*

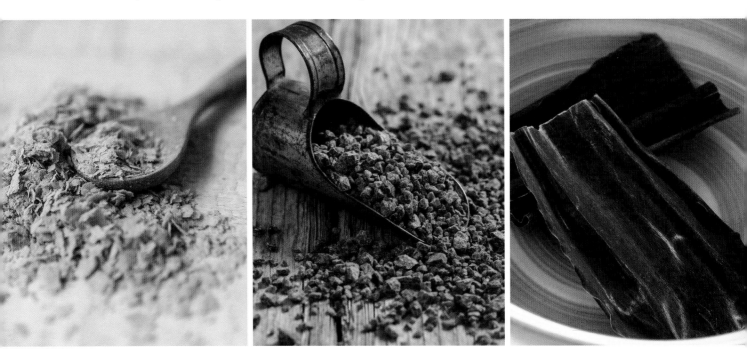

TOFU

Tofu is used quite a lot in this book. It is a wonderfully versatile ingredient as its texture varies according to how much water is pressed out during production, a process that involves soya beans being mashed, cooked and then pressed. Then, and this stage is actually similar to making mozzarella or cottage cheese, a coagulant is added to the pressed-out liquid, which separates into liquids and solids. The solids are tofu. Sometimes the solids are further pressed to make firmer varieties of tofu.

Extra-firm is the most common type of tofu, and often comes in a plastic tray surrounded by water. Extra-firm tofu is a very popular ingredient in vegan cooking because it has a chewy, meaty texture that works well in stews and curries that traditionally use meat. What's more, it absorbs flavours well and can even be marinated. There are many other uses, too: you can attain a delicious crust on the tofu if you place some kitchen paper and a couple of books on top, to press even more water out, and then dust it in cornflour (cornstarch), semolina or polenta and shallow or deep-fry it.

The second most common type is silken tofu, which is very soft, silky and delicate. Unlike firm tofu, it comes in small cardboard boxes and has a very long shelf life. Confusingly, silken tofu has its own variations: soft silken, firm silken, extra-firm silken, etc. In my experience the differences are small and all work fine for a recipe that states 'silken tofu'. Silken tofu is often used for sauces, and can be sliced into delicate cubes and added to soups and stews at the last minute.

VITAL WHEAT GLUTEN AND SEITAN

Vital wheat gluten (or gluten flour) can be used to make some intriguing vegan recipes. It can be purchased in health food stores or online, and is made by washing the starch away from normal wheat flour, leaving behind the protein-rich part of the flour – the gluten.

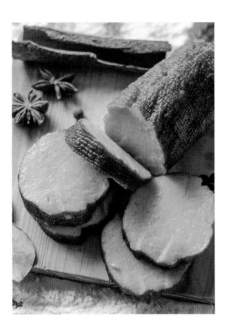

Seitan (pictured above), is an ancient meat-alternative pioneered by Chinese and Japanese Buddhists, made by mixing vital wheat gluten flour with water and boiling the resultant dough. Seitan has the toughest, chewiest, most meat-like texture of all meat-alternatives. Any vegan fried chicken recipe will make use of seitan, including those sold by the new and in-vogue vegan fried chicken outlets and pop-ups.

Vital wheat gluten can also be used to boost the protein in bread or add extra chewiness to bagels.

TEXTURED VEGETABLE PROTEIN (TVP)

TVP is the protein extracted from soya beans. It comes dried, in chunks or with a similar appearance to puffed rice, and is found in large supermarkets and health food stores, probably next to the dried lentils and beans or in the free-from section. You can use it as a high-protein, low-fat meat or mince (ground meat) replacement by rehydrating it in boiling water for about 15 minutes.

'Meat-free mince' products are normally around 97 per cent TVP and found in the frozen foods aisle. I would recommend buying these over dry TVP as manufacturers add a couple of flavourings such as barley malt extract, yeast extract and spices that make it taste quite similar to minced (ground) beef. These use already rehydrated TVP and so don't require soaking in boiling water.

JACKFRUIT

A very large fruit native to South India, jackfruit has a stringy, fibrous texture that, when harvested unripe before it is sweet, makes a very good pulled pork or chicken substitute. Just make sure you buy a can of young 'green' jackfruit in brine rather than ripe jackfruit in syrup, for savoury dishes such as the Jumbo Jackfruit Burritos or Jackfruit Caesar Salad on pages 98 and 94. You can buy it in Asian supermarkets and online.

AQUAFABA

Aquafaba is, bizarrely, the name for the liquid in canned chickpeas. Someone, somehow, discovered that it can be whipped up like egg whites, so you can make vegan meringues, mayonnaise and mousses with it! It is not a storecupboard essential, exactly, but you are likely to come across it in vegan recipes. As you probably stock canned chickpeas, you will already have it to hand.

Below *canned jackfruit.*

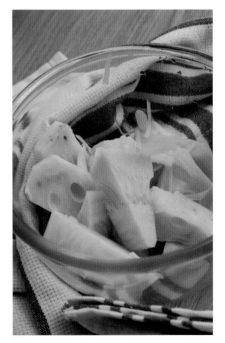

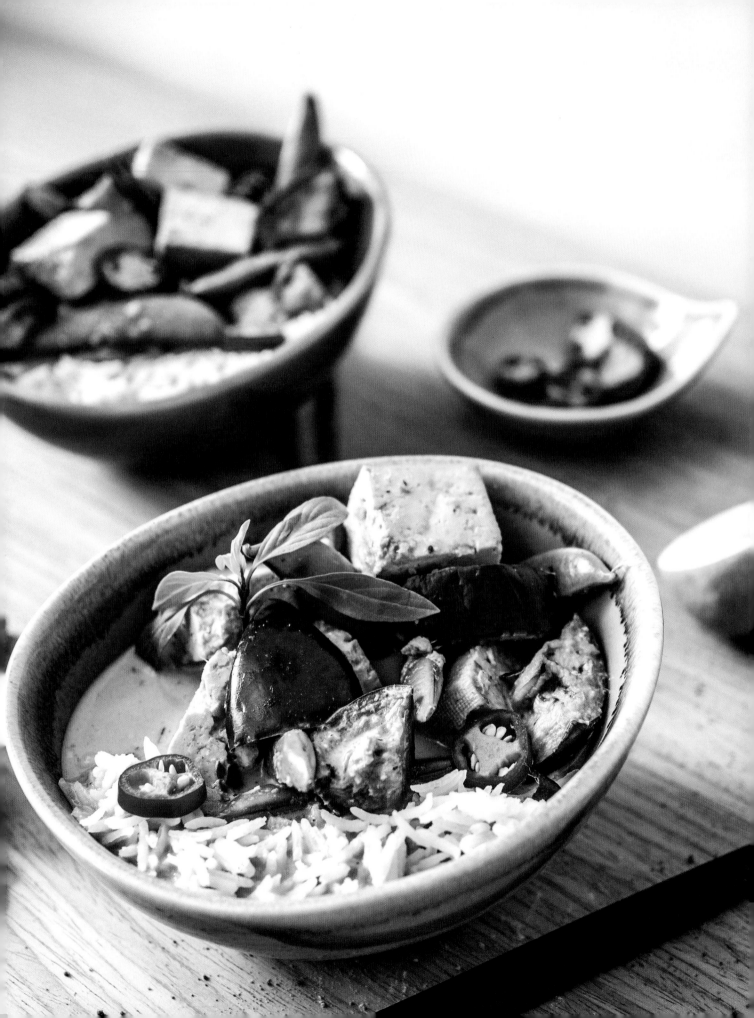

VEGANISE YOUR FAVOURITE DISHES

If a recipe in a magazine catches your eye, you see something on a TV cooking show, or just have a craving for a dish you grew up with, but don't really have a clue how to go about veganising it, you're in the right place. Sometimes the process is straightforward – substituting dairy milk for plant-based milk, for instance – but sometimes you may need a workaround. When baking, for example, cocoa powder, mashed banana and flaxseed gel have the same binding action as eggs (see page 30).

MEATY MEALS

In stews and curries, such as beef casserole or chicken korma, you have a few options. The easiest one is to buy ready-made meat alternatives such as Quorn or supermarket own-brand versions. Quorn often uses eggs and milk proteins, but the company brought out a vegan range in 2016. The technology has come a long way, and the difference between using Quorn vegan meat-free pieces instead of chicken in a stew or pie is nearly indistinguishable. The delightfully named soya chunks work well in stews, too, as they rehydrate, become chewy, and soak up the sauce.

Second, you could use extra-firm tofu. It's healthy, high in protein and widely available, and if you press the water out has a chewy, meaty texture. It is particularly good in Asian dishes such as Thai Green Curry (opposite).

A third option is to try seitan or tempeh, both of which can sometime be quite difficult to find (though they are increasingly available). These are delicious, meaty, savoury products that are very high in protein.

Lastly, you could rely on Mother Nature and use the meatiest vegetables out there: portobello mushrooms or aubergines (eggplants). Portobello mushrooms work well in a stir-fry instead of beef, especially once they

> ### VEGAN GRAVY
> *Peel and finely chop a banana shallot or small onion and fry in a splash of olive oil until golden. Add 5 rehydrated porcini mushroom pieces, with their stock, leaves from 1 sprig of thyme and 60ml/4 tbsp red wine and stir while the wine bubbles. Add a 28g/1oz onion gravy pot, 500ml/17fl oz/generous 2 cups boiling water and stir until the stock has dissolved. Strain if you wish, and serve in a jug.*

shrink and toughen as their water evaporates. Aubergines, cut into cubes, skewered, marinated and then cooked on a barbecue, also have an almost meat-like texture.

Rich stocks are often a fundamental part of meat stews. With time and care you can make a vegan stock that is just as complex and flavoursome. Mushrooms and soy sauce are important as they're naturally high in glutamic acid, the chemical responsible for umami (savoury flavours). See the recipe for good vegetable stock on page 33.

Making a tasty gravy is a little tricky, but can be done. A great start is to fry an onion and then add a good quality vegan stock like 'gravy pot'. Add to that a few rehydrated porcini mushrooms, a splash of red wine, herbs such as thyme and

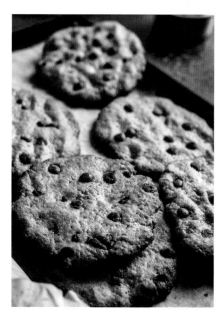

rosemary, and dilute with boiling water.

Burgers, sausages and meatballs can easily be made vegan by using beans instead of meat, seasoning them with spices such as paprika and cumin, and using breadcrumbs and ground flaxseeds/linseeds to bind it all together.

Alternatively, you could make the burgers – and the sausages or meatballs for that matter – out of meat-free mince, which normally consists of textured vegetable protein (TVP). You just need to mix it with your chosen sausage spices, binder and some sautéed aromatics and form it into burgers, sausages or meatballs, as in the 'Meatballs', Mash & Gravy recipe on page 119. Some mainstream supermarkets make an excellent, extremely cheap, vegan mince that you can find in the frozen section. Incidentally, ready-made vegan meatballs are also very good.

You'll be pleased to hear there is a delicious, natural, healthy and unprocessed substitute to pulled pork. Young 'green' jackfruit (find out more about what it is on page 25) has a remarkably similar texture to pulled pork: fibrous, stringy and a little chewy. If you cook it in BBQ sauce, you'll barely notice the difference.

Speaking of pork, bacon is another surprisingly easy meat to substitute. You can use a marinade of smoked paprika, soy sauce, maple syrup, ground black pepper and liquid smoke to flavour

Left *Peanut butter chocolate chip cookies use flaxseeds as a binding agent, (page 140).*

cassava, rice paper or seitan strips, then grill (broil) or fry them up in a good amount of oil, and voilà: crispy bacon. In addition, you can buy quite good ready-made fake bacon ('fakon'). For bacon 'bits', you could fry crumbled coconut chips that have had a good soak in the aforementioned marinade.

You may be wondering how you can possibly replace meals where meat is the main part of the dish, Sunday lunch, for example, or steak and chips on a Friday? Admittedly, these are the hardest meals to veganise, though you can make a pretty realistic steak with seitan, which is sinewy and tough – just like the real thing. Adding paprika and tomato paste to the vital wheat gluten flour mixture used to make the seitan would even create a 'bloody' effect. You can buy ready-made seitan steaks from some health food stores. Another alternative is a nut roast, for which you will find a thousand recipes online, when you add all the 'trimmings' this becomes just as satisfying as a roast meal that features chicken or beef.

MEALS WITH FISH

Similar to meat, if the fish is in a dish, then it is easier to make vegan than if it is the dish, e.g. a fillet of salmon.

A few well-known recipes can be veganised very successfully. Tuna's chewy, chunky texture in a classic tuna mayo can be replicated with mashed chickpeas and made convincing with the addition of lemon juice, red onion, ketchup, corn, salt and ground black pepper – as in the Chickpea 'Tuna' Mayo Sandwich, pictured bottom left, recipe on page 63.

Vegan 'Fish' Cakes (see page 113) are surprisingly realistic: nori sheets (the seaweed used for sushi), white pepper, spring onions (scallions), lemon juice and tomato ketchup all come together with mashed potatoes and chickpeas to make a surprisingly fishy product. Throw toasted ground flaxseeds/linseeds into the mix, which have an abundance of omega-3 oils and so produce a remarkably seaside-y aroma, and you've got yourself some serious fishcakes.

Even Britain's beloved fish and chips can be made vegan. Extra-firm tofu has a similar texture to haddock and cod: fairly delicate with some resistance. Covered in batter and deep-fried, it is an excellent alternative. In fact, a bespoke 'Tofu 'n' Chips' shop has recently opened in Bristol in the west of England, and the dish can be found on menus elsewhere in the UK. To have a go yourself, see the Tofu Fish 'n' Chips recipe on page 114.

For breaded fish products, such as fish fingers, fillets or nuggets, frozen 'fishless' or 'fish-style' fingers, as well as nuggets and other breaded products are readily available in many supermarkets and wholefood stores. They are very convenient for a weeknight oven-dinner – and surprisingly evocative of your childhood favourites.

MEALS RICH IN DAIRY

Many classic recipes require a rich, thick, dairy-based sauce. Cauliflower cheese, pasta bake, lasagne ... the list goes on. Pleasingly, you can make all of these vegan with a little know-how.

For a classic white sauce, the best solution is to take a literal approach: baking block margarine for the butter and soya milk for the dairy milk. The result may not be quite as rich, but it will work. Perhaps a splash of soya cream could raise the vegan version's game.

When dairy cheese is actually incorporated in the sauce, for instance

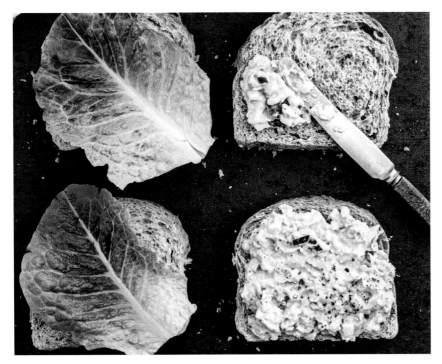

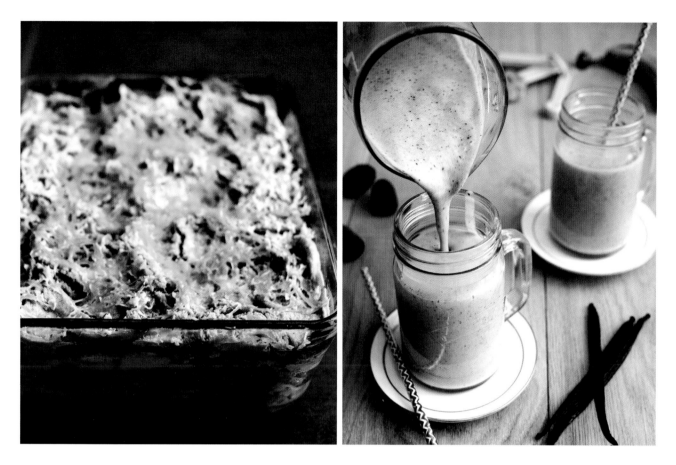

in macaroni cheese recipes, a different approach is often taken: cashew nuts. These nuts, soaked for a few hours in water and blended, create a creamy, thick mixture that, combined with nutritional yeast, makes an excellent cheese sauce.

But what about the cheesy, crispy topping? You could buy vegan mozzarella-style cheese or vegan pizza shreds, or some people stick to a topping made of dried breadcrumbs, and perhaps a few hazelnuts, crushed tortilla chips or crisps (US potato chips), which will still make a delicious crust, despite the absence of any real or fake cheese. This line of thought applies to pizza, too; vegan cheese is an option, but some prefer to pile silky roasted vegetables straight on to an aromatic tomato sauce, and skip the 'cheese' altogether.

You could also experiment with other techniques: the lasagne recipe on page 108, pictured above, uses puréed celeriac and olive oil for the 'béchamel'. The nacho 'cheese' sauce on page 73 is surprisingly, almost questionably, similar to real nacho cheese, and uses potatoes, carrots and liberal amounts of oil and nutritional yeast, instead of dairy.

There are thousands of drinks and desserts that rely heavily upon dairy. If you want to make a whipped or double (heavy) cream-based dessert, you have a few options. You can use coconut cream (sometimes called creamed coconut), or the top of a can of full-fat coconut milk that has separated into cream and water, to make an excellent vegan coconut whipped cream (see box).

Ice cream is easy to substitute since coconut, almond and soya milk-based ice creams are just as delicious as dairy. All mainstream supermarkets seem to stock at least one – Swedish Glace is widely available. You could also just use sorbet. Any kind of smoothie is possible with nut-based milks, such as the Date and Banana Smoothie (above) on page 36.

Fermented dairy products, such as buttermilk and yogurt, have a variety of uses. A buttermilk alternative can be made by adding 15ml/1 tbsp lemon juice to 250ml/8fl oz/1 cup unsweetened

---

COCONUT WHIPPED CREAM

Refrigerate a 400ml/14oz can of full-fat coconut milk overnight – the cream will separate from the liquid. Chill a bowl and electric whisk attachments for an hour before making the cream. Remove the hardened coconut cream from the can (keep the separated liquid for smoothies) and whisk with the chilled electric whisk until fluffy (not too long, or it will separate). Add 25g/1oz/¼ cup icing (confectioners') sugar and whisk again until creamy. Use immediately or refrigerate (it will harden further in the fridge).

soya milk and leaving it to thicken for 10 minutes.

It is possible to make your own vegan yogurt by fermenting soya or coconut milk with a pack of vegan bacterial cultures, but it's hardly the easy option – how many people make their own dairy yogurt? Bought vegan yogurts have come a long way, to the point that they are affordable, have a great consistency, and even my dad will eat them.

Cream cheese and sour cream alternatives can both be made by blending cashew nuts that have been soaked in water overnight with onion powder and nutritional yeast for the former and lemon juice for the latter. See the box for a recipe. The brand Tofutti make excellent vegan versions of both, and other own-brand vegan cream cheeses will do for baking (as in Lemon No-bake Cheesecake on page 139), although I wouldn't recommend you spread them on a bagel...

For baking, substituting butter for baking block margarine is a simple and effective solution. You can also substitute coconut oil, as it's also solid at room temperature (which is important in baking), but it's more expensive and will

QUICK BANANA ICE CREAM

Peel, chop and freeze 4 large, very ripe bananas overnight. Blend thoroughly in a high-powered blender or food processor with 30ml/2 tbsp caster (superfine) sugar or another sweetener (optional – the bananas may be sweet enough already) and 30ml/2 tbsp plant-based milk. Sparingly add more plant-based milk if it gets stuck while blending. Serve immediately or re-freeze for 20–30 minutes if the warmth from the blender has melted the bananas.

change the flavour of whatever you're making. Oil will generally work as a direct replacement for butter, especially in cakes, but the resultant texture will be slightly different – if you do this, make sure you use a refined, neutral-tasting oil such as sunflower since others, such as sesame or olive oil, will give your baked goods a very distinct flavour!

EGGS AS AN INGREDIENT OR AS A MEAL ON THEIR OWN

Eggs need veganising in a few ways, as of course non-vegans use them not only as a binding agent, but also a standalone meal in themselves.

When eggs are used to bind foods together, you have a few options. Both ground flaxseeds/linseeds and chia seeds absorb water and thicken into a binding gel. Broadly speaking, flaxseeds/linseeds work better than chia seeds. One 'flax egg' (see box) can replace one real egg in recipes for cakes, cookies, muffins and even savoury foods such as vegan meatballs and burgers. They can also be used to thicken smoothies. Chia seeds are more suitable for raw dishes, such as 'chia pudding' and 'chia jam', or baked goods such as pancakes where the rise and texture aren't as important as in, say, a sponge cake.

You could also purchase a bespoke egg-replacer, which are mainly made of starches and natural gums and work well in cakes – just add a little more fat to make up for the missing egg yolks. And in some recipes – e.g. banana bread or pancakes – mashed banana will work like a charm.

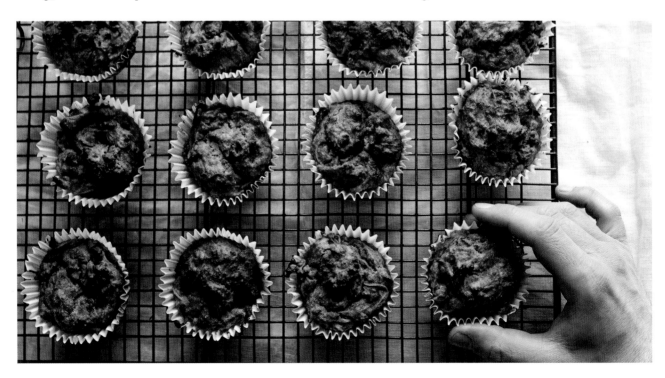

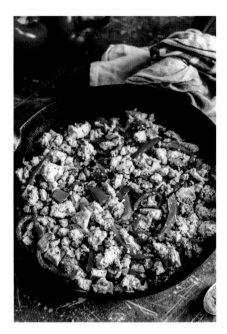

Eggs are sometimes used as a pastry glaze, or wash. This can be substituted with a mixture of soya milk and maple syrup – a 3:1 soya milk to maple syrup ratio is a good rule of thumb.

It may sound impossible to replace eggs when they're used as a meal in themselves. Indeed, some dishes are impossible, such as a boiled egg (that is, until eggs can be grown in labs...). However, options do exist for other egg dishes, most of which rely upon tofu, gram (chickpea) flour and sometimes a type of Indian black salt called kala namak (see page 24).

Tofu scramble is the most well-known alternative. Extra-firm tofu is slightly tough and rubbery, but rather crumbly and – loosened with a little plant-based milk – imitates the texture of scrambled eggs well. Adding a little ground turmeric gives a lovely golden-yellow hue, and throw some sweated onions and (bell) peppers in there and you've got yourself a delicious brunch. See Tofu Scramble (pictured above) on page 50.

You can give the tofu scramble, or any egg-imitation dish for that matter, a greatly increased eggy flavour and smell with the addition of kala namak. This ingredient is high in sulphur compounds, meaning that it smells and even tastes like eggs. Just add 2.5ml/½ tsp to your dish when you add the other spices, and refrain from using any normal salt.

Spanish omelettes can be veganised more easily than lighter egg dishes as they rely on potatoes for structure. Combine with some gram flour for its colour, slightly nutty flavour, and absence of gluten, and you've got yourself a decent Spanish omelette. A similar idea can be applied to frittatas.

Vegan omelettes make use of gram flour, too, often in conjunction with silken tofu, which lightens the texture and adds creaminess. Quiches work in a similar way but have a shortcrust pastry casing. And while pastry is on your mind, that isn't a problem at all, as most store-bought pastry uses oil and so

is vegan anyway, or you can easily make it yourself by replacing the butter with baking block margarine.

If you are going to add vegetables to your frittata, omelette (Spanish or otherwise) or quiche, make sure they are fully cooked beforehand so there's no excess moisture that will result in a watery, steamed-rather-than-baked dish to ruin your morning.

And lastly, eggs are traditionally used to make mayonnaise and, of course, mayonnaise derivatives: aioli, tartare sauce, ranch dip, etc. Mayonnaise is my absolute favourite condiment, so I was relieved to find that very good vegan versions exist, which you can buy in health food stores, and, pleasingly, some mainstream supermarkets, which have recently started stocking the best (in my opinion) vegan mayo available – Vegenaise by Follow Your Heart. It's also easy to make your own – see page 32, pictured below. Whichever you use, the door to dips, coleslaws, creamy pasta and potato salads is wide open.

Lastly, aquafaba – the liquid from a can of chickpeas – can be used to make vegan meringues, as it whips up just like egg whites.

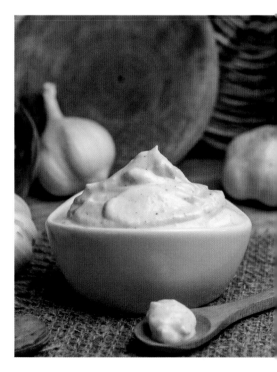

VEGAN CONDIMENTS

It's hugely reassuring to have a few standby vegan substitutes that you can quickly whip up and keep in the fridge. Once you have a delicious mayo or satay sauce in your repertoire, being vegan seems much more feasible!

VEGAN MAYONNAISE/AIOLI

Makes: 250ml/9fl oz/1 cup

120ml/4fl oz/½ cup unsweetened soya milk, at room temperature
5ml/1 tsp Dijon mustard
15ml/1 tbsp lemon juice
15ml/1 tbsp cider vinegar
2.5ml/½ tsp caster (superfine) sugar
2.5ml/½ tsp fine salt
1.25ml/¼ tsp ground black pepper
120ml/4fl oz/½ cup vegetable oil
15ml/1 tbsp garlic purée (optional, if making aioli)

1 Put all the ingredients, apart from the oil and garlic, in a blender or food processor, or a bowl if using a stick blender. Blitz until smooth.

2 With the motor running, pour the oil in as slowly as possible – not so slowly that it drips in but in the slowest possible stream. If using a stick blender, add 15ml/1 tbsp at a time between short blitzes until none is left. This helps the mayo to thicken up.

3 If making aioli, add the garlic purée and blitz again.

4 Transfer to airtight containers and keep in the fridge. The mayo will thicken as it chills.

TARTARE SAUCE

Makes: 250ml/8fl oz/1 cup

225g/8oz/1 cup vegan mayonnaise
2 medium gherkins (pickles), finely chopped
30ml/2 tbsp capers, drained and roughly chopped

15ml/1 tbsp finely chopped fresh dill
15ml/1 tbsp lemon juice
7.5ml/½ tbsp cider vinegar 2.5ml/ ½ tsp Dijon mustard
2.5ml/½ tsp caster (superfine) sugar
2.5ml/½ tsp fine salt
1.25ml/¼ tsp ground black pepper

1 Put all the ingredients in a medium bowl and stir well. Transfer to an airtight container and keep in the fridge for up to two weeks.

2 Serve with 'fish' cakes on page 113 or tofu 'fish' and chips on page 115.

VERSATILE VEGAN PESTO

Makes: 225ml/8fl oz/1 cup

50g/2oz/⅓ cup almonds, pine nuts, cashew nuts, walnuts or pistachio nuts
100g/3¾oz/2 packed cups fresh basil, parsley, rocket (arugula) or baby spinach
1 medium garlic clove, finely chopped or crushed
45ml/3 tbsp lemon or lime juice
about 1.25ml/¼ tsp fine salt
75ml/2½fl oz/⅓ cup virgin olive oil

1 Dry-fry the nuts in a medium frying pan over a medium-high heat for 5–10 minutes, until toasted and fragrant. Keep your eye on them and toss regularly so they don't burn.

2 Put the chosen herb, nuts, garlic, lemon or lime juice and salt in a food processor or blender. Pulse until roughly blended. You could also use a bowl and stick blender or a mortar and pestle, in which case add the herbs in small batches.

3 Drizzle the oil in slowly, with the motor running. If using a stick blender or mortar and pestle, add the oil 15ml/1 tbsp at a time in between blending or pounding.

4 Stop to scrape down the sides, pulse again, then taste and add more salt if necessary. Pulse or pound again.

5 Use immediately or transfer to an airtight container. It freezes well. Toss with pasta for a quick and easy supper.

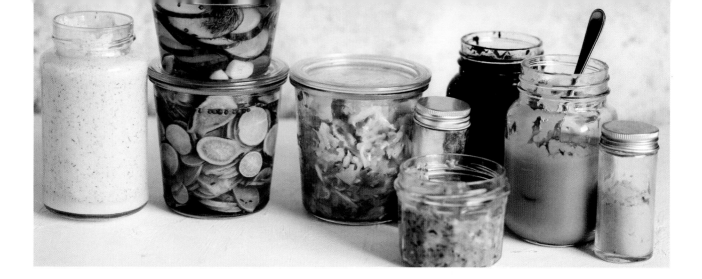

ASIAN PEANUT SAUCE

Makes: 225ml/8fl oz/1 cup

85g/3½oz/⅓ cup smooth peanut butter
30ml/2 tbsp soy sauce
30ml/2 tbsp lime juice or juice of 1 lime
15ml/1 tbsp maple syrup
5ml/1 tsp garlic paste

5ml/1 tsp ginger paste
10ml/2 tsp toasted sesame oil
45ml/3 tbsp water
a pinch of cayenne pepper

1 Put all the ingredients in a blender or food processor and blitz to a

smooth, runny sauce. Equally, you could do this in a medium bowl, using a stick blender or a small whisk.

2 Use as a stir-fry sauce, or as a dipping sauce with raw vegetable crudités or fried tofu.

CAESAR/RANCH DRESSING

Makes: 1 large or 2 small jars

300g/11oz silken tofu, drained
30ml/2 tbsp vegan mayonnaise
45ml/3 tbsp nutritional yeast
1 garlic clove, crushed
15ml/1 tbsp extra virgin olive oil

zest and juice of ½ lemon (about 22.5ml/1½ tbsp juice)
15ml/1 tbsp cider vinegar
5ml/1 tsp Dijon mustard
3.75ml/¾ tsp fine salt
2.5ml/½ tsp caster (superfine) sugar
1.25ml/¼ tsp ground black pepper

1 Put all the ingredients in a blender or food processor and blitz until smooth. You could also put everything in a bowl and use a small whisk.

2 Store in the fridge and use to dress any kind of salad.

PROPER HOMEMADE VEGETABLE STOCK

Makes: 1 litre/1¾ pints/4 cups

60ml/4 tbsp neutral vegetable oil
250g/9oz chestnut or button (white) mushrooms, halved
1 large onion, roughly chopped
2 medium carrots, roughly chopped
2 celery sticks, roughly chopped
8 whole black peppercorns
4 garlic cloves, sliced
3 fresh or dried bay leaves
5 sprigs of fresh thyme
10 medium (5g/⅛oz) dried porcini mushroom pieces
2.5ml/½ tsp fine salt

1 In a large pan or stockpot, heat 30ml/2 tbsp of the oil over a high heat. Add the halved mushrooms and fry for about 10 minutes so they get a good amount of colour.

2 Add the remaining oil along with the onion, carrots, celery and peppercorns. Fry for 5 minutes, still over a high heat.

3 Add the garlic and fry for 1–2 more minutes, until golden, then add the bay leaves, thyme, porcini mushrooms and salt along with 1 litre/1¾ pints/ 4 cups water.

5 Bring to a boil, then reduce to a low simmer, cover and leave to cook for about 1 hour.

6 Strain the stock through a colander into a large bowl. Press the vegetables down with the back of a wooden spoon to release as much liquid and flavour as possible.

7 Discard all the vegetables and store the stock in airtight containers. It freezes well. Use for all kinds of soups, pasta sauces, stews and curries in place of a stock cube.

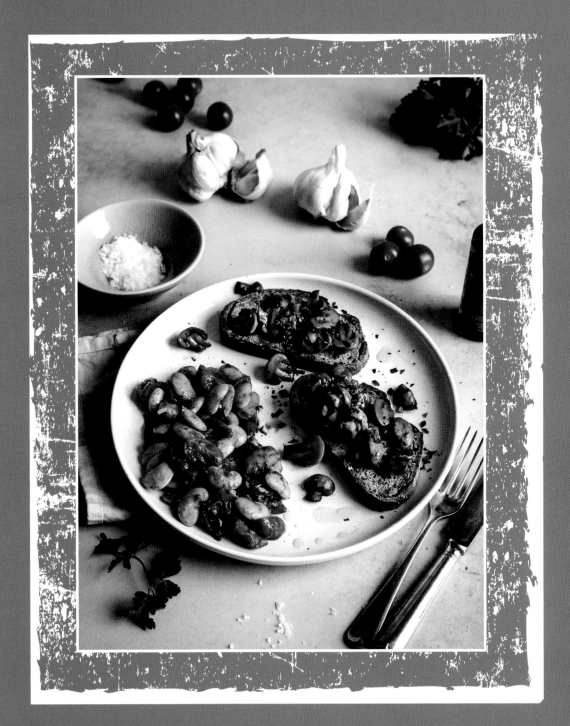

BREAKFAST AND BRUNCH

DATE & BANANA SMOOTHIE

Serves: 1
Equipment: blender
Prep time: 5 minutes
Cooking time: none

Individually, all the ingredients in this smoothie are super healthy, and yet somehow they come together to taste almost indulgently delicious – certainly greater than the sum of the parts. Like an excellent football team, much unlike any I've ever been a part of...

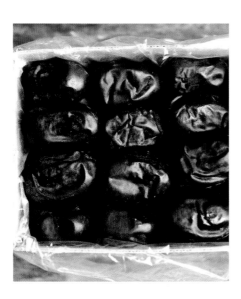

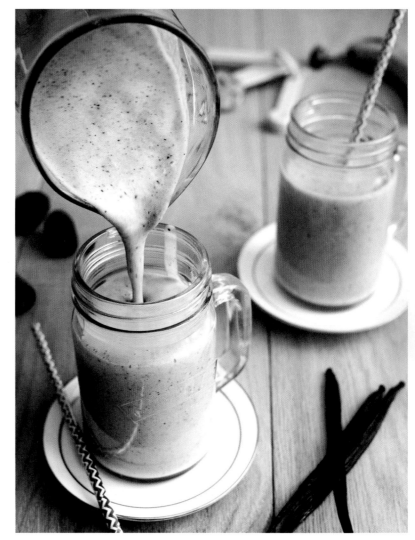

4 large (or 6 small) Medjool dates, pits removed
1 large ripe banana, chopped
45ml/3 tbsp pumpkin seeds
22.5ml/1½ tbsp peanut butter (crunchy or smooth)
1.25ml/¼ tsp ground cinnamon
1.25ml/¼ tsp vanilla extract
3 large ice cubes
200ml/7fl oz/scant 1 cup unsweetened soya milk

SUBSTITUTE INGREDIENTS
Dates: *double the quantity of normal dates, pitted*
Pumpkin seeds: *Hemp or sunflower seeds*
Peanut butter: *Nut butter of choice*
Soya milk: *other plant-based milk of choice*

1 Put all the ingredients into a blender.

2 Blitz until smooth, adding more soya milk if the smoothie is too much of a thickie for your tastes.

ALMOND BUTTER OVERNIGHT OATS

Makes: 2 jars
Equipment: jam jars or cylindrical airtight containers with lids
Prep time: 5 minutes, plus overnight soaking
Cooking time: none

This is an excellent way of preparing a fuelling, healthy breakfast ahead of time. Having a jar of these to grab on your way out of the house will help you avoid how my mornings often pan out: drinking coffee on an empty stomach and visibly shaking until lunchtime – not a good look.

115g/4oz/1¼ cups rolled oats
250ml/8fl oz/1 cup rice milk or other plant-based milk
10ml/2 tsp maple syrup
1.25ml/¼ tsp ground cinnamon
pinch of salt
15ml/1 tbsp smooth almond butter

Toppings (optional):
fresh fruit, e.g. banana, berries
seeds or chopped nuts
soya or coconut yogurt

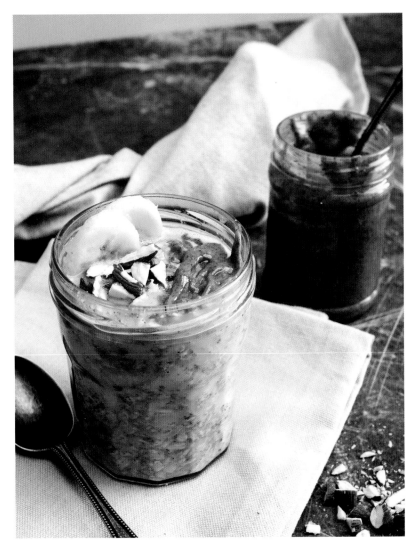

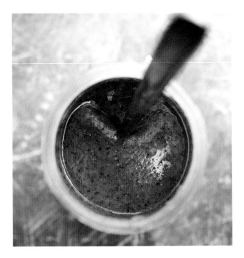

1 Divide the oats equally between two empty jam jars or cylindrical tupperware containers.

2 Add half the remaining ingredients to each jar or container, stir thoroughly and seal.

3 Chill in the fridge overnight and they'll be ready to eat the next morning. Add toppings just before eating, if you want to.

NUT & SEED GRANOLA

Granola is the ultimate flexi-recipe; feel free to substitute your favourite dried fruit and nuts, or get creative and use spelt, barley or rye flakes instead of oats. I like a dash of salt in mine for contrast (akin to salted caramel) but have left it optional.

Makes: 1kg/2¼lb
Equipment: large bowl, 1–2 large baking trays, airtight containers
Prep time: 10 minutes
Cooking time: 20–30 minutes

450g/1lb/4 cups jumbo oats
75g/3oz/½ cup blanched almonds, roughly chopped
50g/2oz/⅓ cup Brazil nuts, roughly chopped
50g/2oz/⅓ cup pumpkin seeds
65g/2½oz/⅓ cup buckwheat groats
25g/1oz/⅓ cup coconut chips
60ml/4 tbsp golden (light corn) syrup
45ml/3 tbsp maple syrup
30ml/2 tbsp neutral vegetable oil
0.6ml/⅛ tsp fine salt (optional)
150g/5oz/1 cup flame raisins
50g/2oz/⅓ cup chopped dried figs
50g/2oz/⅓ cup chopped dried apricots

1 Preheat the oven to 170°C/340°F/Gas 3½.

2 Thoroughly mix the oats, nuts, seeds, groats and coconut chips with the golden syrup, maple syrup, oil and salt (if using) in a large bowl.

3 Spread the mixture out in a single, shallow layer on a large baking tray (you may need two trays).

4 Bake in the oven for 20–30 minutes, turning the mixture over with a wooden spoon halfway through the cooking time, until golden brown. Check regularly to make sure it's not burning.

5 Once golden brown, turn the oven off and leave the granola inside with the oven door ajar slightly to dry out for 30 minutes.

6 Remove from the oven, mix in the dried fruit and leave to cool completely. Store in airtight containers.

SUBSTITUTE INGREDIENTS

Jumbo oats: *rye flakes or spelt flakes*
Blanched almonds and Brazil nuts: *macadamia or cashew nuts*
Pumpkin seeds: *sunflower seeds*
Golden (corn) syrup: *rice or agave syrup*
Raisins: *sultanas*
Dried figs: *prunes*
Dried apricots: *dried cranberries or dried cherries*

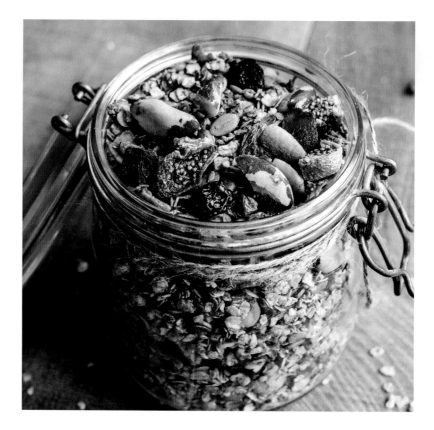

FRUIT, YOGURT & GRANOLA POTS

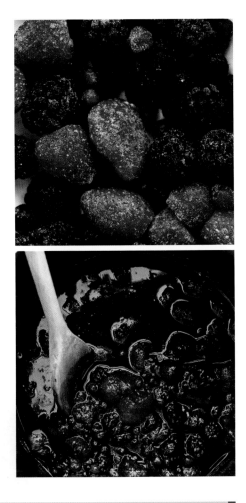

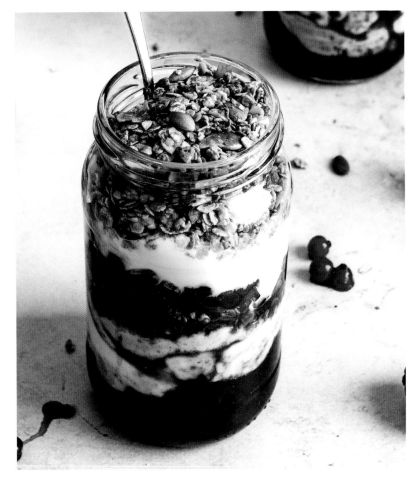

Fruit compote should really be harder, or more expensive, to make than it is. Chuck some frozen berries, sugar and a small splash of water in a pan, lid on and away you go. If you have a large batch of the compote and some vegan yogurt in the fridge, and some suitable granola in the cupboard, you have breakfasts-to-go in just 5 minutes.

Makes: 4 pots
Equipment: medium pan with a lid, jam jars or pots with lids
Prep time: 5 minutes
Cooking time: 45 minutes

1kg/2¼lb mixed frozen fruit, such as raspberries, blueberries, blackberries

50g/2oz/¼ cup caster (superfine) sugar

500g/1¼lb plain soya yogurt or coconut milk yogurt

250g/9oz/2 cups granola (check it doesn't contain honey, or make your own), or vegan muesli

1 Put the frozen fruit, sugar and 30ml/2 tbsp water into a medium pan over a low heat. Put the lid on and cook for 45 minutes, stirring halfway through the cooking time. Once finished, remove from the heat, uncover and leave to cool completely.

2 Spoon a layer of the fruit compote into the bottom of each jar or pot.

3 Add a layer of yogurt and then a handful of granola.

4 Repeat this layering process until the jars or pots are nearly full. Put the lid on and keep in the fridge until required.

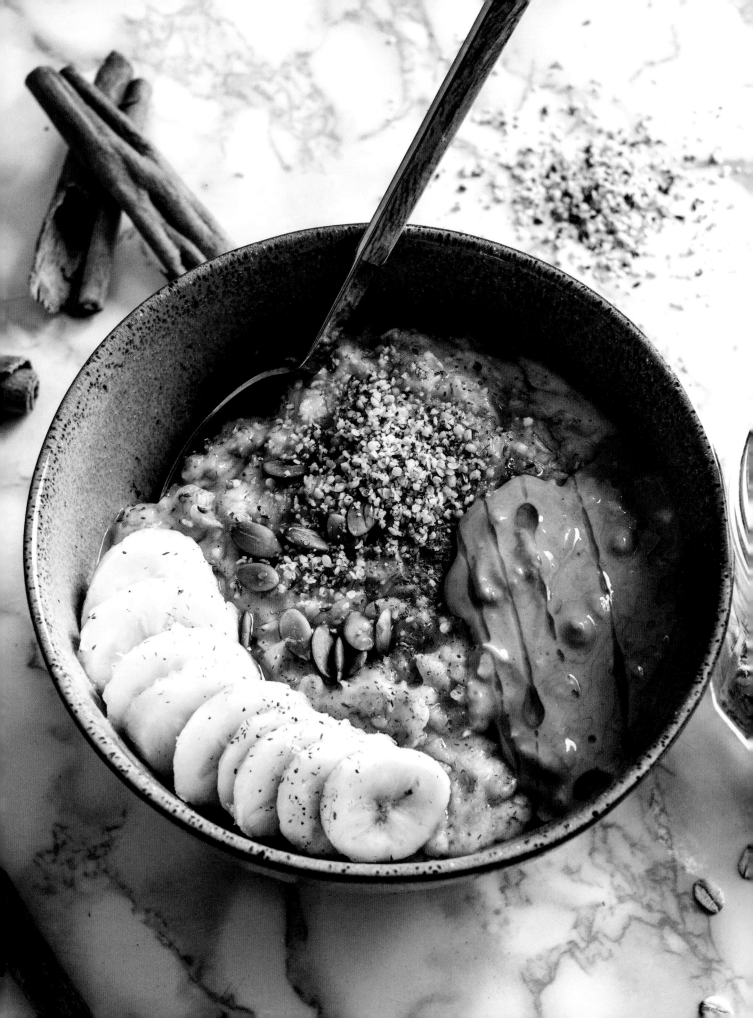

PROTEIN-PACKED PORRIDGE

What better way to set you up for the day than a hefty shot of protein (without using powder), healthy fats and complex carbohydrates to boot? This nourishing porridge is really simple to throw together, and a joy to eat. Tuck in.

Serves: 1
Equipment: small pan
Prep time: 5 minutes
Cooking time: 5 minutes

60g/2½oz/⅔ cup rolled oats
300ml/½ pint/1¼ cup unsweetened soya milk
pinch of fine salt
pinch of ground cinnamon
1 small banana, sliced
15ml/1 tbsp crunchy peanut butter
10ml/2 tsp hemp seeds
15ml/1 tbsp pumpkin seeds
7.5ml/1½ tsp maple syrup

1 Put the oats and soya milk in a small pan, bring to a boil, then reduce the heat to medium-low.

2 Stir in the salt and cinnamon. Cook for 4 minutes, stirring slowly and frequently, until thick.

3 Ladle into a bowl and top with the sliced banana, peanut butter, hemp seeds, pumpkin seeds and maple syrup.

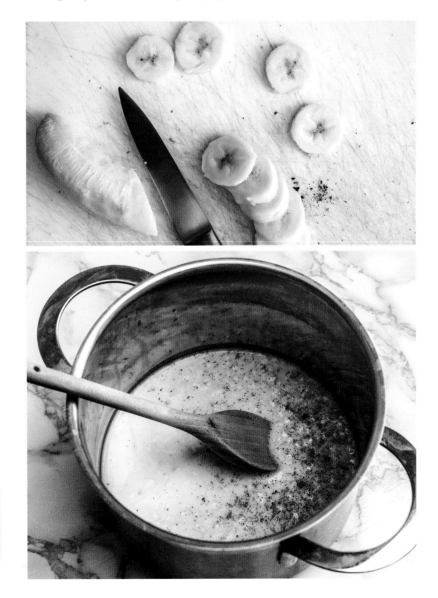

SUBSTITUTE INGREDIENTS
Soya milk: *any plant-based milk*
Peanut butter: *almond or cashew butter*
Hemp seeds: *chia or sesame seeds*
Pumpkin seeds: *sunflower seeds*

HEALTHY BREAKFAST MUFFINS

These muffins rival porridge for the coveted set-you-up-for-the-day breakfast award. They are made with wholemeal flour and oats, naturally sweetened by grated apples and banana, and have a root vegetable snuck in. Don't expect huge, billowing muffins, as they're weighed down by all those superfoods, but they are in no way stodgy.

Makes: 16 muffins
Equipment: 2 muffin trays, 16 muffin cases, food processor or blender, large bowl, grater, medium bowl
Prep time: 15 minutes
Cooking time: 25–30 minutes

For the dry ingredients:
90g/3½oz/1 cup rolled oats
250g/9oz/generous 2 cups plain wholemeal (whole-wheat) flour
1.25ml/¼ tsp fine salt
2.5ml/½ tsp ground ginger
1.25ml/¼ tsp ground cinnamon
7.5ml/1½ tsp baking powder

For the wet ingredients:
2 medium or large apples, preferably a sweet variety
2 medium ripe bananas, roughly chopped
250ml/8fl oz/1 cup plant-based milk of choice
120ml/4fl oz/½ cup neutral vegetable oil
175g/6oz sweet potato or carrot

1 Preheat the oven to 180°C/350°F/Gas 4. Line a couple of muffin trays with the muffin cases.

2 Blitz the oats in a food processor or blender to a fine oat flour. Mix the oat flour with the other dry ingredients in a large bowl and set aside.

3 Chop the apples in half and cut out the cores. Finely chop or grate the apples using a food processor or grater (you don't need to peel them). Transfer to a medium bowl. No need to wash up the food processor as you will use it again.

4 Mash the bananas into the grated apples, then whisk in the plant-based milk and oil. Finely chop or grate the sweet potato or carrot using a food processor or grater (you don't need to peel them).

5 Stir the grated sweet potato or carrot and the apple-banana mixture into the dry ingredients until all the flour is hydrated. Try to mix as little as possible. Don't worry if it's a little lumpy.

6 Spoon the mixture into the muffin tray cases and bake for 25–30 minutes, rotating the trays halfway through the cooking time if the muffins are unevenly browning. Cover loosely with foil if they brown too quickly.

7 Insert a skewer into a muffin to check if they are cooked. If the skewer comes out clean, they are done. Let the muffins cool in the tray for 5 minutes, then transfer them to a wire rack and leave until completely cool.

8 Store in an airtight container, transferring this to the fridge the next day to keep the muffins fresh. Alternatively, you can freeze them.

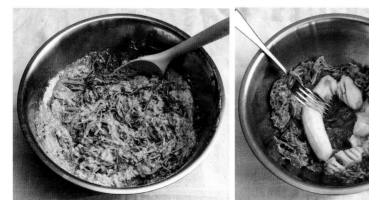 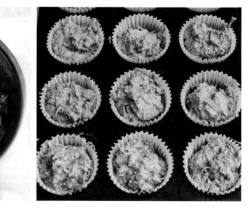

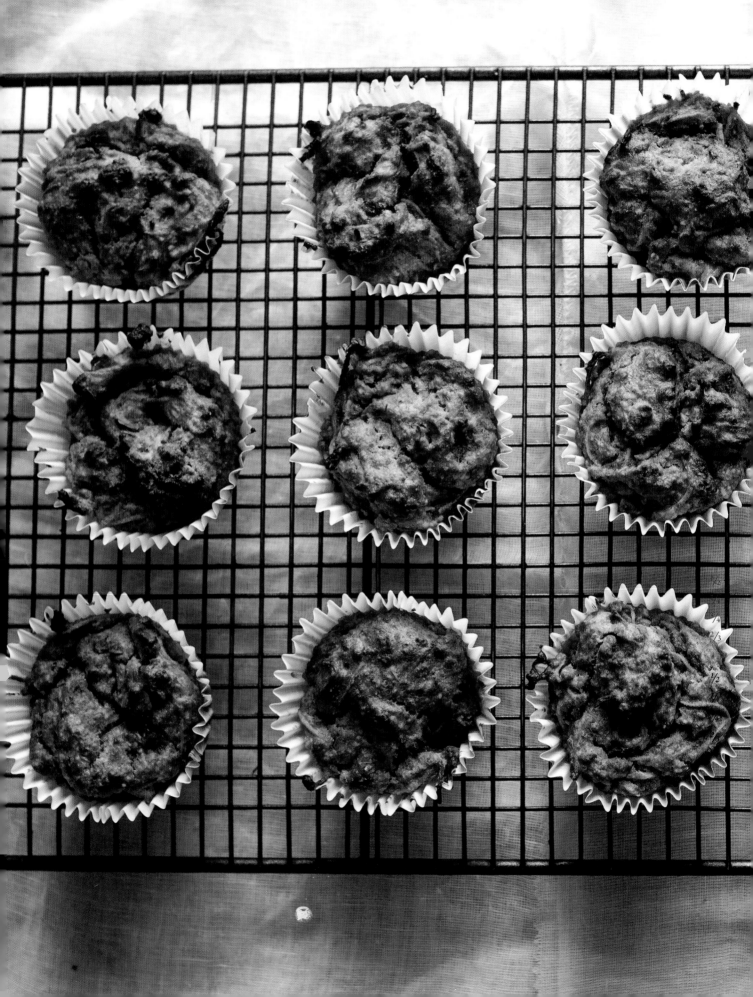

4-INGREDIENT PEANUT BUTTER HOTCAKES

Peanut butter is my desert island ingredient. Without doubt. I eat it every day and slip it into my meals whenever I can. Porridge? – better with peanut butter. Salad? – better with an Asian peanut dressing. Baked tofu? – better with peanut satay sauce. It produces the goods again with these simple little hotcakes.

Makes: 4 small pancakes (serves 1)
Equipment: food processor, large non-stick frying pan
Prep time: 5 minutes, plus standing time of at least 15 minutes
Cooking time: 5–10 minutes

50g/2oz/scant ½ cup rolled oats
½ medium-large ripe banana (65g/2½oz peeled weight), chopped
15ml/1 tbsp smooth peanut butter*
15ml/1 tbsp neutral vegetable oil

To serve (optional):
blueberries and maple syrup
or strawberries and coconut yogurt
or banana and chocolate chips

1 Blitz the oats in a food processor to a fine oat flour. Add the banana, peanut butter and 120ml/4fl oz/½ cup water to the food processor. Blitz again until smooth. Leave the batter to stand for at least 15 minutes or up to 2 hours.

2 Heat the oil in a large non-stick frying pan over a medium heat. Add one-quarter of the batter per pancake. You may have room to fry them all at once in your frying pan – if not, fry them in batches. Fry for 2–3 minutes until golden brown, flip over with a spatula, and fry the other side for 1–2 minutes, until also golden.

3 Transfer the pancakes to a plate, then cook the remaining batter if there is any. Top with whatever you fancy – suggestions: blueberries and maple syrup, strawberries and coconut yogurt, banana and dark chocolate chips.

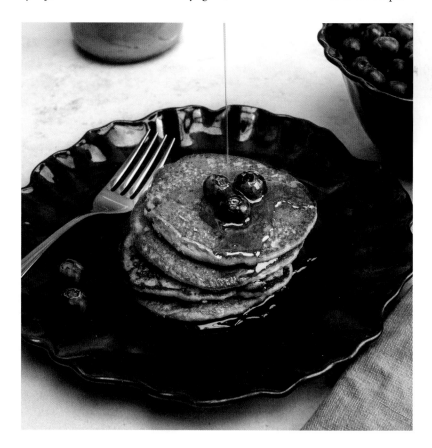

* If you're using unsweetened, unsalted peanut butter, you may want to add a little sugar and salt to the pancake mix.

BUBBLE & SQUEAK

Serves: 2
Equipment: large bowl, large non-stick frying pan
Prep time: 10 minutes
Cooking time: 7 minutes

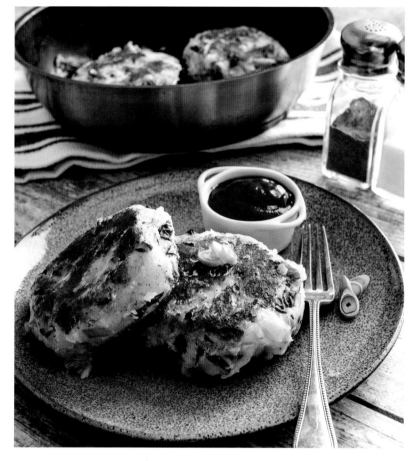

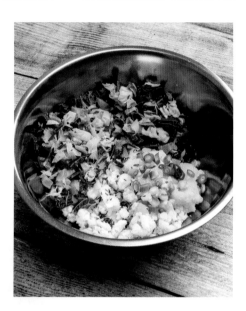

400g/14oz leftover mashed, roasted or boiled potatoes

200g/7oz leftover cooked cabbage or Brussels sprouts, roughly chopped

2 spring onions (scallions), whites and greens, sliced

2 sprigs of fresh thyme, leaves only

2.5ml/½ tsp fine salt

1.25ml/¼ tsp ground black pepper

flour, for dusting

45ml/3 tbsp olive oil

To serve (optional):
tomato ketchup

As a child, the name Bubble and Squeak scared me. I don't quite know why – perhaps I found the onomatopoeic description of the dish frightening. I've since got over it.

1 If you are using leftover boiled or roasted potatoes, put them in a large bowl and roughly mash them, leaving a few chunks. Otherwise, put the mashed potato in a large bowl.

2 Add the cabbage, spring onions, thyme, salt and ground black pepper and mix well.

3 Divide the potato mixture into four. Lightly flour your hands and form the portions into balls. Gently flatten each ball to make round, 2.5cm/1in-thick potato cakes.

4 Heat the olive oil in a large non-stick frying pan over a medium heat. Fry the potato cakes for 4 minutes on one side, then gently flip them and fry for 3 more minutes on the other side, until golden and crispy. Serve 2 cakes per person with a dollop of ketchup on the side, if you like.

FULL ENGLISH BREAKFAST

Of the, say, ten possible ingredients in a classic Full English, many are already, or can easily become, vegan: baked beans, hash browns, grilled mushrooms, etc. A generous amount of oil is needed to bring the meal up to 'greasy spoon' standards, so don't be shy with it. To me, the breakfast isn't 'Full' without sliced white bread and a pot of strong tea.

Serves: 2
Equipment: large roasting tray, small pan, medium frying pan
Prep time: 10 minutes
Cooking time: 25 minutes

400g/14oz waxy potatoes, cubed
4 vegan sausages
2 large beefsteak tomatoes, cut in half horizontally
90ml/6 tbsp neutral vegetable oil
5ml/1 tsp fine salt
4 large portobello mushrooms, stalks removed
a little ground black pepper
400g/14oz can baked beans
2 slices of white bread
10ml/2 tsp vegan margarine

To serve (optional):
tomato ketchup or brown sauce

1 Preheat the grill (broiler) to medium-high and grease a large roasting tray.

2 Put the potatoes in a small pan, cover with water and bring to a boil. Turn the heat down to a simmer and cook for 8 minutes. Drain, then transfer to paper towels or a clean dish towel and set aside.

3 Meanwhile, put the sausages and tomatoes on the greased roasting tray, tomatoes cut-side up. Drizzle over 30ml/2 tbsp of the oil and sprinkle with 2.5ml/½ tsp of the salt, then grill (broil) for 6 minutes. Add the mushrooms, upside down, to the roasting tray and grill for 6 minutes more, or until everything is cooked and nicely browned. Turn off the grill, leaving the tray inside to keep everything warm.

4 Heat the remaining 60ml/4 tbsp oil in a medium frying pan over a medium-high heat. Add the parboiled potatoes and fry, turning regularly, for 10 minutes. Season with the remaining 2.5ml/½ tsp salt and a little ground black pepper.

5 Meanwhile, heat up the baked beans in a bowl in the microwave or in a small pan on the hob. Just before the potatoes are ready, toast the bread and brew some tea.

6 Spread the toast with margarine and slice it in half diagonally. Serve the toast with 2 mushrooms, 2 tomato halves, 2 sausages and some potatoes and beans for each person, along with a dollop of ketchup and brown sauce, if you like.

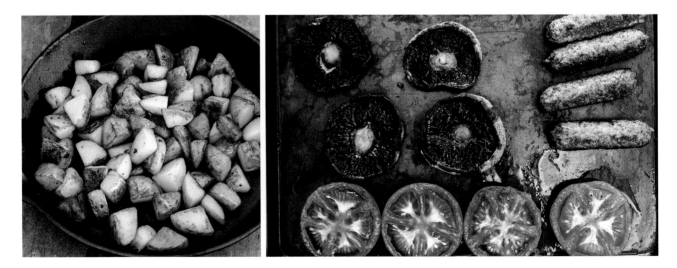

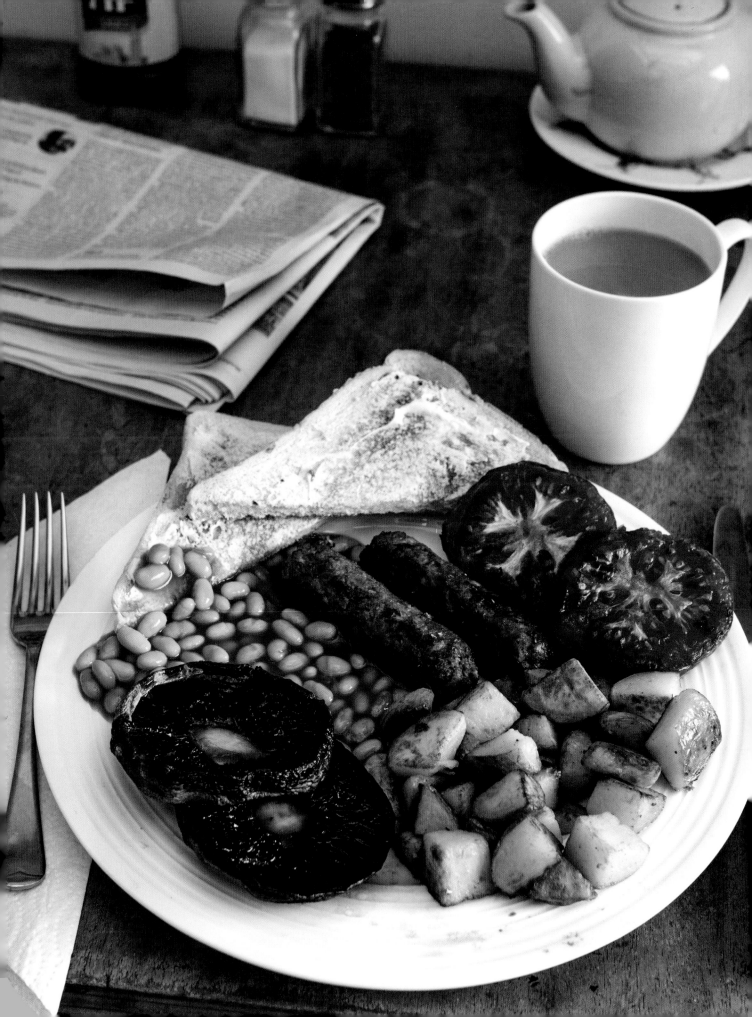

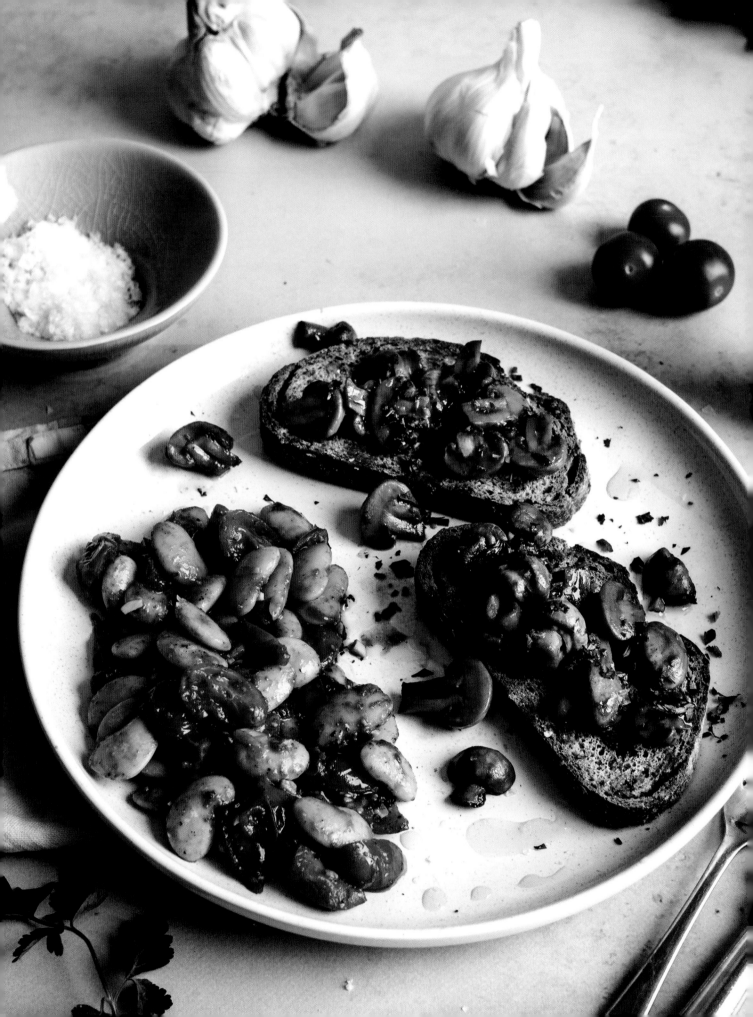

MUSHROOMS & BIG BEANS ON SOURDOUGH

Some friends of mine made a dish similar to this using fresh cherry tomatoes instead of canned ones, resulting in a fresher, more vibrant sauce for the beans that I preferred. The soy and brown sauces give the mushrooms an unusual, rich, salty-sweet flavour. Sourdough bread adds a hearty chew underneath, but is not essential; you can use whatever bread you happen to have.

Serves: 2
Equipment: 2 medium frying pans
Prep time: 10 minutes
Cooking time: 25 minutes

75ml/5 tbsp olive oil
4 garlic cloves, finely chopped
10 cherry tomatoes, quartered
15ml/1 tbsp tomato paste
5ml/1 tsp caster (superfine) sugar
2.5ml/½ tsp fine salt
1.25ml/¼ tsp ground black pepper, plus extra for serving
400g/14oz can butter (lima) beans, drained and rinsed
250g/9oz button (white) mushrooms, halved
15ml/1 tbsp soy sauce
10ml/2 tsp brown sauce
2–4 thick slices of sourdough bread
15ml/1 tbsp extra virgin olive oil
15ml/1 tbsp finely chopped parsley

1 Heat 45ml/3 tbsp of the olive oil in a medium frying pan over a medium heat. Add half of the garlic and sauté for 3 minutes, then add the tomatoes and tomato paste, stir, and cook for 7 more minutes.

2 Roughly mash the tomatoes with the back of a wooden spoon. Add the sugar, salt and ground black pepper, then stir in the butter beans. Cook for 5 more minutes.

3 Meanwhile, heat the remaining 30ml/2 tbsp olive oil in another medium frying pan over a medium-high heat. Add the remaining garlic, fry for 1–2 minutes, then add the mushrooms and cook for 10 minutes.

4 Stir the soy sauce and brown sauce into the mushrooms and cook for 3 more minutes.

5 Meanwhile, toast the bread, drizzle it with oil and put in on plates. Pile on the mushrooms and serve beans to the side. Season with extra black pepper and sprinkle over the parsley.

SUBSTITUTE INGREDIENTS
Cherry tomatoes: *200g/7oz canned tomatoes, chopped*
Butter beans: *cannellini beans*
Soy sauce: *tamari sauce*

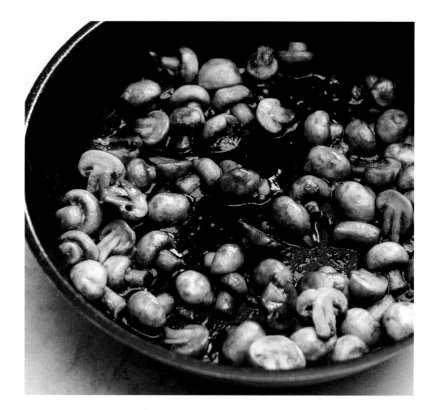

TOFU SCRAMBLE WITH ONIONS & PEPPERS

Tofu is remarkably versatile, and quite unique. Depending on how much it is pressed, it can be smooth and silky like double cream or firmer, like scrambled eggs, as is the case here. I like my scrambled tofu with sautéed bell peppers and onions and seasoned with a good grinding of black pepper. The scramble works well as a quick supper dish too.

Serves: 2
Equipment: kitchen paper or clean dish towels, heavy weight, large frying pan
Prep time: 10 minutes, plus 30 minutes pressing
Cooking time: 25 minutes

400g/14oz extra-firm tofu, drained
45ml/3 tbsp olive oil
½ medium onion, chopped
1 red (bell) pepper, seeded and sliced
2.5ml/½ tsp ground turmeric
2.5ml/½ tsp yeast extract
10ml/2 tsp nutritional yeast
2.5ml/½ tsp fine salt or kala namak
1.25ml/¼ tsp ground black pepper, plus extra to serve (optional)
2 thick slices of wholemeal (whole-wheat) bread
10ml/2 tsp vegan margarine or extra virgin olive oil

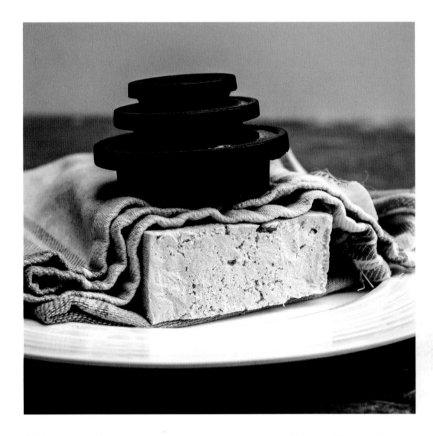

1 Place several layers of kitchen paper, or a couple of clean dish towels, on a plate. Put the tofu on the towels and cover with more paper/dish towels. Place a heavy object, such as a book or a heavy pan, on top to press the water out of the tofu. Leave to drain for at least 30 minutes. If you're short of time, press down on the heavy object to get as much water out of the tofu as possible.

2 Heat the oil in a large frying pan over a medium heat. Add the onion, red pepper, turmeric and yeast extract to the pan and sauté for 15 minutes.

3 Crumble the pressed tofu into the pan, aiming for a scrambled-egg consistency. Stir in the nutritional yeast, salt or kala namak and ground black pepper. Sauté for 10 minutes.

4 Toast the bread, spread with margarine or olive oil and put it on to two plates. Top with the tofu scramble and season with extra ground black pepper, if you like.

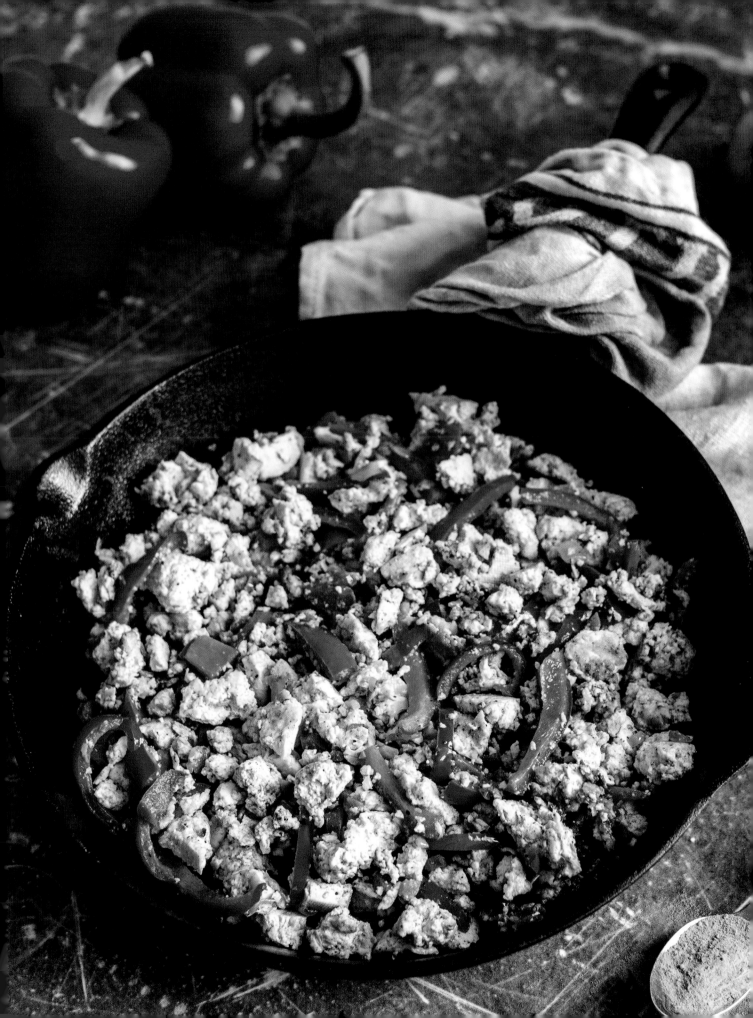

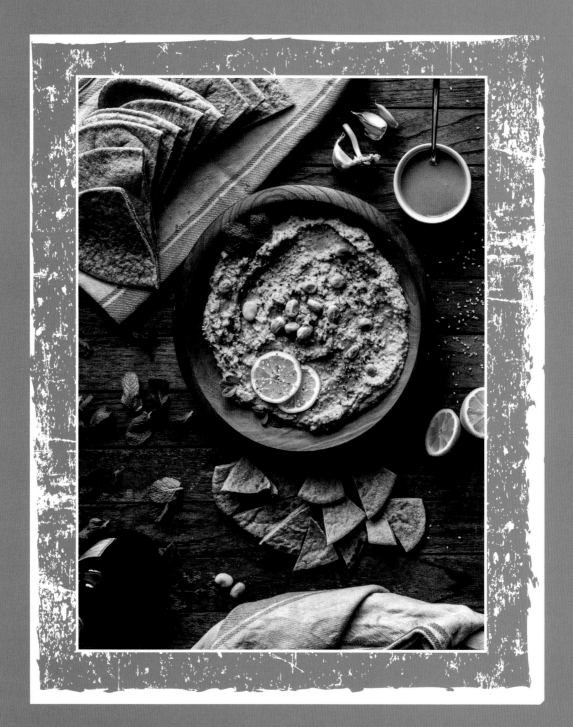

SNACKS AND SIDES

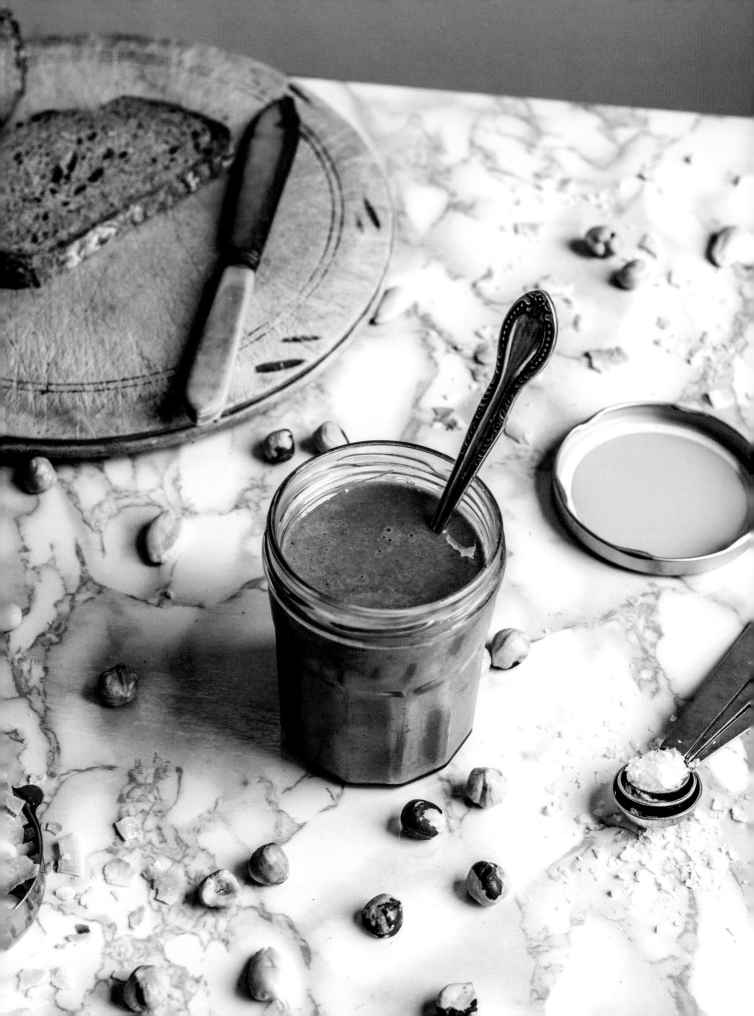

ROASTED ALMOND, COCONUT & HAZELNUT BUTTER

Occasionally, just *occasionally*, I feel like branching out and away from my beloved peanut butter. I don't stray too far away – I don't want it to be offended – but we need a little break from each other once in a while. I go as far as this almond and hazelnut butter, which is delectably creamy and has an additional flavour dimension from a handful of coconut flakes.

Makes: 250g/9oz/1¼ cups
Equipment: large baking tray, food processor or powerful blender, jar or airtight container
Prep time: 10 minutes, plus 15 minutes cooling
Cooking time: 12 minutes

200g/7oz/1⅓ cups blanched almonds
80g/3¼oz/½ cup blanched hazelnuts
20g/¾oz/¼ cup coconut flakes
5ml/1 tsp coconut oil
2.5ml/½ tsp soft light brown sugar
1.25ml/¼ tsp fine sea salt

1 Preheat the oven to 180°C/350°F/Gas 4. Spread out the almonds and hazelnuts on a large baking tray and toast for up to 12 minutes, adding the coconut flakes to the tray for the final 2 minutes. Watch carefully as they burn quickly.

2 When the nuts and coconut chips are golden brown, remove from the oven and leave to cool for about 15 minutes.

3 Once cool, put the almonds, hazelnuts, coconut flakes and coconut oil in a food processor or powerful blender and blend for 3–6 minutes, or until the oil releases and the mixture becomes creamy.

4 Scrape the mixture down the sides of the bowl, then add the sugar and salt and blend again for 15 seconds.

5 Decant into a jar or airtight container. No need to refrigerate. If when you come to use it you find the nut butter has separated and the oil has floated to the top, just stir it thoroughly with a fork.

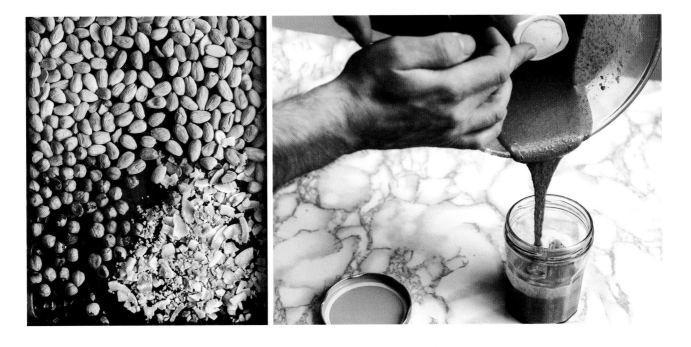

POWER BARS

These are extremely useful for when you're on the go. What's more, they're lower in sugar than any bars you'll find at the supermarket, as well as being packed full of vitamins, minerals and healthy fats, and a healthy dose of plant-based protein.

Makes: 12 bars
Equipment: 25 x 20 x 3cm/10 x 8 x 2in roasting tray or baking tin (pan), small bowl, medium baking tray, food processor or jug blender, large bowl, heatproof bowl or small pan, large wooden spoon or spatula
Prep time: 10 minutes, plus 15 minutes soaking
Cooking time: 40 minutes

45ml/3 tbsp chia seeds
a little neutral vegetable oil, for greasing
40g/1½oz/⅓ cup blanched hazelnuts, chopped
50g/2oz/⅓ cup pumpkin seeds
250g/9oz/generous 2½ cups rolled oats
22.5ml/1½ tbsp cacao nibs
115g/4oz/⅔ cup chopped dates
65g/2½oz/½ cup hemp seeds
30ml/2 tbsp smooth almond butter
75ml/5 tbsp maple syrup
0.6ml/⅛ tsp fine salt
30ml/2 tbsp coconut oil

1 Mix the chia seeds with 135ml/9 tbsp water in a small bowl and set aside to soak for 15 minutes. They will absorb the water and turn into a gel.

2 Meanwhile, preheat the oven to 180°C/350°F/Gas 4. Grease the roasting tray or baking tin with a little oil.

3 Spread out the hazelnuts, pumpkin seeds and half the oats on a medium baking tray and bake for 10 minutes, until golden brown.

4 Use a food processor or jug blender to blitz the remaining oats to a coarse flour. Transfer to a large bowl, then add the toasted hazelnuts, pumpkin seeds and oats, as well as the chia seed gel, cacao nibs, chopped dates, hemp seeds, almond butter, maple syrup and salt.

5 Melt the coconut oil in a heatproof bowl in the microwave (it will only need 20–30 seconds) or in a small pan on the hob and add to the bowl.

6 Mix everything together very thoroughly with a large wooden spoon or spatula so the almond butter is well incorporated.

7 Transfer the mixture to the greased roasting tray or baking tin and firmly press flat.

8 Bake for 30 minutes, then remove from the oven and leave to cool completely (this will take a couple of hours).

9 Slice into 12 bars using a sharp knife while it is still in the tray or tin. Carefully remove the bars and store in an airtight container in the fridge. They can also be frozen.

SUBSTITUTE INGREDIENTS
Hazelnuts: *almonds or Brazil nuts*
Cacao nibs: *vegan dark chocolate chips*
Raisins: *dried figs or apricots*
Hemp seeds: *sunflower seeds or pine nuts*
Almond butter: *smooth peanut butter*
Maple syrup: *agave or date syrup*

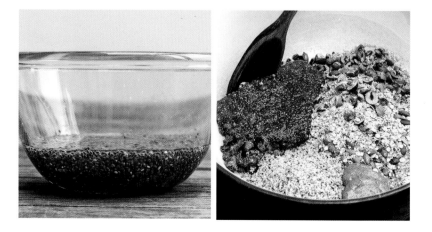

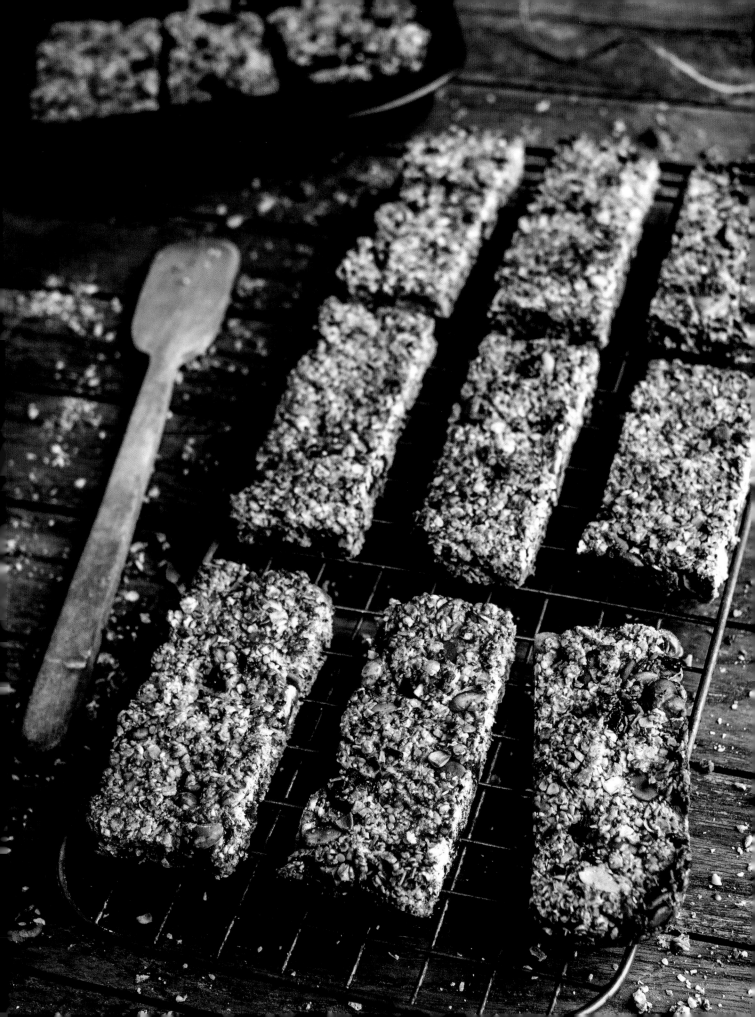

CASHEW TZATZIKI

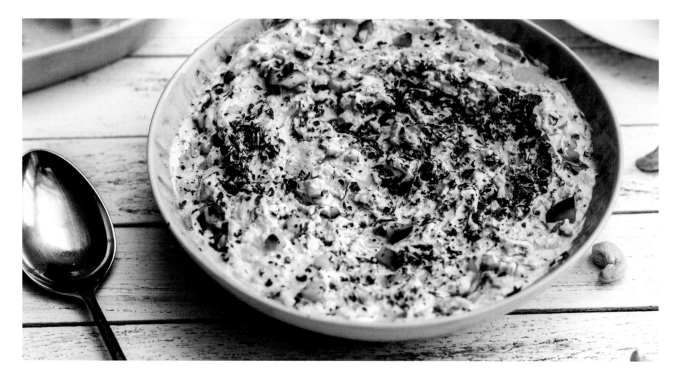

Cashews, soaked overnight in water and then blitzed, blend to a rich, creamy consistency, which makes a brilliant base for a vegan tzatziki that is delicious served as part of a mezze feast, or just as a snack with some crackers, carrots and tomatoes.

Makes: 750ml/1¼ pints/3 cups
Equipment: strainer, powerful blender or food processor, or mixing bowl and stick blender
Prep time: 5 minutes, plus at least 3 hours soaking and 30 minutes chilling
Cooking time: none

225g/8oz/2 cups unroasted, unsalted cashew nuts
45ml/3 tbsp lemon juice
2 medium garlic cloves, crushed
3.75ml/¾ tsp fine salt
2.5ml/½ tsp ground black pepper
½ medium cucumber, very finely chopped (it will seem like too much, but is not)
2 packed handfuls (about 15g/½oz) of fresh mint leaves, finely chopped
a drizzle of extra virgin olive oil and an extra grind of black pepper, to garnish

1 Soak the cashew nuts in a bowl of water for a minimum of 3 hours (overnight is best), although if pressed for time, you could soak them for 2 hours in warm water or just 15 minutes in boiling water. The result won't be as creamy, but it will work.

2 Strain the soaked cashew nuts and rinse well with cold water.

3 Transfer the cashew nuts to a powerful blender and add 120ml/4fl oz/½ cup water. Blitz to a fine, smooth, creamy consistency. You could use a food processor or a bowl and stick blender, but the result won't be as smooth. You may need to scrape down the sides.

4 Add the lemon juice, garlic, salt and ground black pepper and blitz again until smooth. It should have a thick, yogurty consistency. Add a little more water if it is too thick, bearing in mind that it will thicken in the fridge.

5 Transfer to a serving bowl and add most of the cucumber and mint, reserving some for the garnish, then stir through. Chill for at least 30 minutes before serving. Garnish with the reserved mint leaves and tiny pieces of cucumber, a drizzle of olive oil and a good grind of black pepper.

BROAD BEAN HUMMUS

Makes: 425g/15oz/1¾ cups
Equipment: food processor or blender, or mixing bowl and stick blender
Prep time: 5 minutes
Cooking time: none

300g/11oz/1½ cups frozen broad (fava) beans, thawed

37.5ml/2½ tbsp lemon juice

30ml/2 tbsp tahini

1 medium garlic clove, crushed

45ml/3 tbsp finely chopped fresh mint

2.5ml/½ tsp fine salt

90ml/6 tbsp extra virgin olive oil

sesame seeds, smoked paprika and extra olive oil, for garnishing

crackers, vegetable crudités or warm pitta breads, to serve

Elsewhere in this book I state emphatically that peanut butter is my desert island ingredient. Hummus comes a close second. There are plenty of chickpea hummus recipes out there, so here's a little variation that I particularly like. Broad beans make a fresher, more vibrant hummus than chickpeas but are still robust and chunky enough for a thick, substantial dip. To emphasise the fruitiness, there is a higher olive oil-to-tahini ratio than in normal hummus.

1 Put the broad beans, lemon juice, tahini, garlic, mint and salt in a food processor or blender (or a mixing bowl if using a stick blender) and blitz to a rough paste.

2 With the motor running, slowly drizzle in most of the olive oil. If using a stick blender, add 15ml/1 tbsp at a time in between blending in bursts.

3 Transfer to a wide serving bowl, and sprinkle with sesame seeds and a little smoked paprika. Drizzle with a little more olive oil and serve with crackers, vegetable crudités or warm pitta breads.

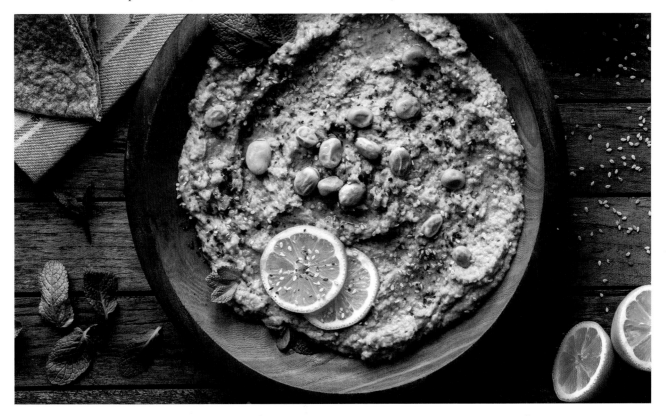

PATATAS BRAVAS

Place a bowl of these crisp, spicy potatoes in the centre of the table and arm friends with a fork or skewer. Equally, take a bowl for yourself, grab a beer from the fridge and stick the TV on. Perfect. There will be leftover sauce, which will be delicious tossed through pasta or roasted chickpeas the next day, or can be portioned up and frozen.

Serves: 4
Equipment: large roasting tray, medium frying pan, jug blender or stick blender
Prep time: 10 minutes
Cooking time: 30 minutes

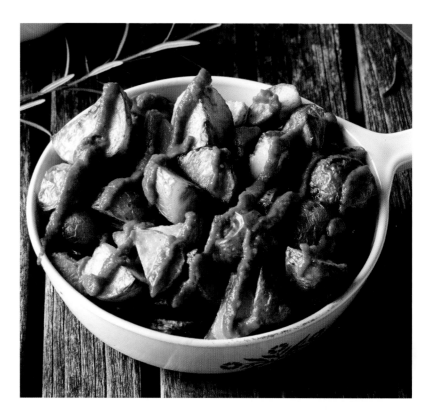

1kg/2¼lb waxy potatoes, chopped into 4cm/1½in cubes
90ml/6 tbsp olive oil
12.5ml/2½ tsp flaky sea salt
1 medium red onion, chopped
1 red (bell) pepper, chopped
4 large garlic cloves, sliced
15ml/1 tbsp smoked paprika
10ml/2 tsp dried oregano
5ml/1 tsp dried rosemary
2.5ml/½ tsp caster (superfine) sugar
a pinch of cayenne pepper
400g/14oz can chopped tomatoes

To serve (optional):
Vegan Aioli (see page 32)

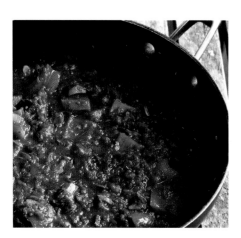

1 Preheat the oven to 200°C/400°F/Gas 6. Put the potatoes in a large roasting tray and toss with 60ml/4 tbsp of the olive oil and 7.5ml/1½ tsp of the salt. Roast in the oven for 30 minutes, shaking halfway through the cooking time.

2 Meanwhile, heat the remaining 30ml/2 tbsp olive oil in a medium frying pan over a medium heat. Add the onion and red pepper and fry for 10 minutes, then add the garlic and cook for 5 more minutes.

3 Stir in the smoked paprika, oregano, rosemary, sugar, cayenne pepper and remaining 5ml/1 tsp sea salt. Cook for 5 more minutes. Add the chopped tomatoes to the pan and cook for 5 more minutes, stirring frequently.

4 Pour the sauce into a jug blender and blitz until smooth, or leave the sauce in the pan and blitz until smooth using a stick blender.

5 Put the roasted potatoes in a wide serving bowl and drizzle with the sauce. Serve immediately with Aioli, if you wish.

PERFECT BASMATI RICE

Before I discovered this technique, I was terrible at cooking rice; it would stick to the bottom of the pan, in an overcooked mush, and somehow still have random hard, uncooked grains. Badly cooked rice can have a significantly detrimental effect on the whole meal, no matter how tasty the other part is. Follow these steps, though, and it'll always be fluffy and delicious!

Serves: 4 as a side
Equipment: bowl, fine-mesh strainer, medium pan with a tight-fitting lid, fork
Prep time: 1 minute, plus 10 minutes standing
Cooking time: 12 minutes

300g/11oz/1½ cups basmati rice
2.5ml/½ tsp fine salt

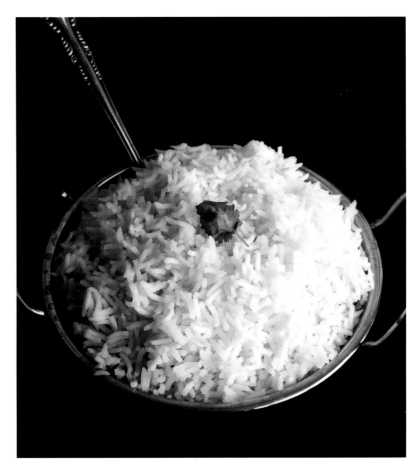

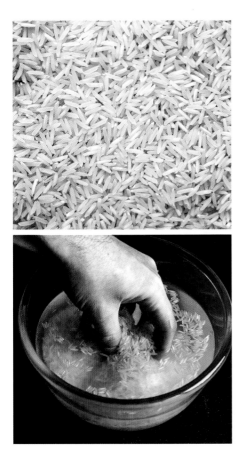

1 Put the rice in a bowl with roughly double the volume of water. Swish it around for 20–30 seconds, until the water is very cloudy. Drain using a fine-mesh strainer.

2 Rinse the rice again under the tap, then transfer it to a medium pan with a tight-fitting lid. Add 550ml/18fl oz/2¼ cups water and the salt, and bring to a boil over a high heat (uncovered). As soon as it boils, turn the heat down to very low, cover with the lid and cook for 12 minutes exactly.

3 Without removing the lid, take the pan off the heat and leave, still covered, for 10 minutes. The rice will finish cooking in the steam trapped inside the pan.

4 Fluff the rice with a fork and serve.

ROASTED VEGETABLE BULGUR WHEAT

This simple dish is perfect to take to a barbecue. Sumac is my favourite spice for its deep purple colour and unexpected citrussy zing, which zips right through the bulgur wheat. Don't skimp on the olive oil; if anything, drizzle more on top. The dish should be fruity, silky and satisfying – not a worthy affair!

Serves: 4 as a side or 2 as a main
Equipment: large roasting tray, foil (optional), pan, large bowl
Prep time: 15 minutes
Cooking time: 30 minutes

1 large aubergine (eggplant), cubed
1 red (bell) pepper, seeded and chopped
1 yellow (bell) pepper, seeded and chopped
1 green (bell) pepper, seeded and chopped
3 courgettes (zucchini), chopped
45ml/3 tbsp olive oil
45ml/3 tbsp red wine vinegar
30ml/2 tbsp dried oregano
5ml/1 tsp sumac
225g/8oz/1¼ cups bulgur wheat
175g/6oz/1 cup Kalamata olives, pitted and halved
22.5ml/1½ tbsp lemon juice
2.5ml/½ tsp fine salt
2 packed handfuls (about 30g/1½oz) fresh parsley, finely chopped
400g/14oz can chickpeas, drained and rinsed (optional)

1 Preheat the oven to 200°C/400°F/Gas 6. Put all the vegetables on a large roasting tray and toss with the oil, vinegar, oregano and sumac.

2 Roast in the oven for 30 minutes, checking after 20 minutes and shaking halfway through the cooking time. Cover loosely with foil if they look like they're beginning to burn.

3 Meanwhile, cook the bulgur wheat in a pan according to packet instructions until just tender. Transfer to a large bowl.

4 Gently mix the roasted vegetables, olives, lemon juice, salt and parsley into the bulgur wheat. Add the chickpeas to make it more substantial, if you like. Serve warm or cold.

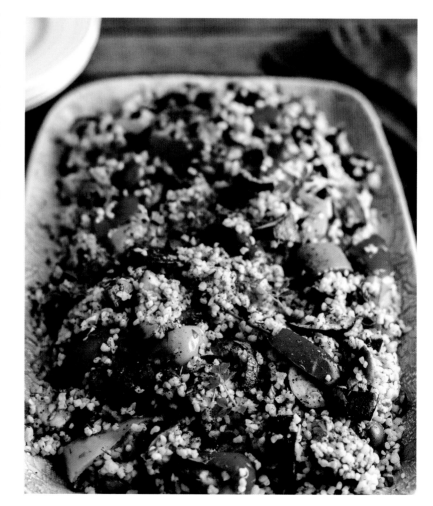

SUBSTITUTE INGREDIENTS
Sumac: *15ml/1 tbsp more lemon juice*
Bulgar wheat: *couscous, farro, freekeh, quinoa – all cooked according to packet instructions*
Parsley: *coriander (cilantro)*

CHICKPEA 'TUNA' MAYO SANDWICH

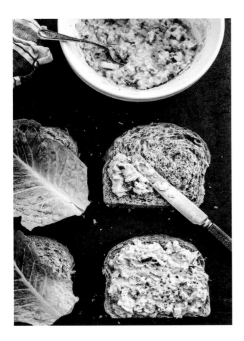

Calling this a tuna sandwich sounds gimmicky, I know, but does it matter if it tastes delicious? I like a drop of Tabasco in my sandwich, and chewy, thickly sliced wholemeal bread, but you can obviously mix it up however you like.

1 Roughly mash the chickpeas with a fork or potato masher in a bowl to a chunky texture.

2 Stir in the corn, red onion, mayonnaise, ketchup, lemon juice and Tabasco sauce, to taste. Taste the mixture and add salt and pepper and extra lemon juice and/or Tabasco until it's just right.

3 Put a lettuce leaf on a slice of bread, then pile on some of the chickpea 'tuna' followed by half the cucumber slices. Close the sandwich with another slice of bread.

4 Repeat for the other sandwich, then slice in half diagonally and store in an airtight container in the fridge if not eating immediately.

Makes: 2 sandwiches
Equipment: fork or potato masher, bowl
Prep time: 5 minutes
Cooking time: none

For the filling:
400g/14oz can chickpeas, drained and rinsed
200g/7oz can corn, drained and rinsed
½ small red onion, finely chopped
60ml/4 tbsp vegan mayonnaise
15ml/1 tbsp tomato ketchup
30ml/2 tbsp lemon juice
a few drops of Tabasco sauce (optional)
1.25ml/¼ tsp fine salt
1.25ml/¼ tsp freshly ground black pepper

To serve:
2 small romaine or cos lettuce leaves, 8 slices of cucumber
4 thick slices wholemeal bread

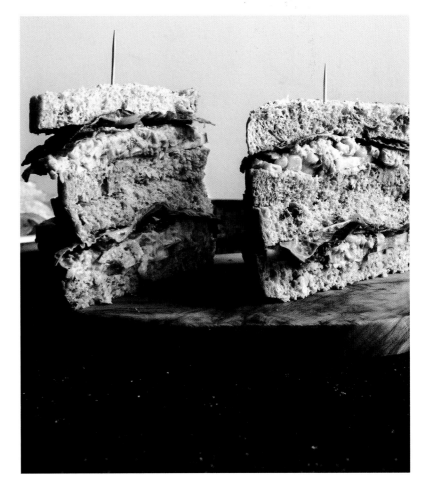

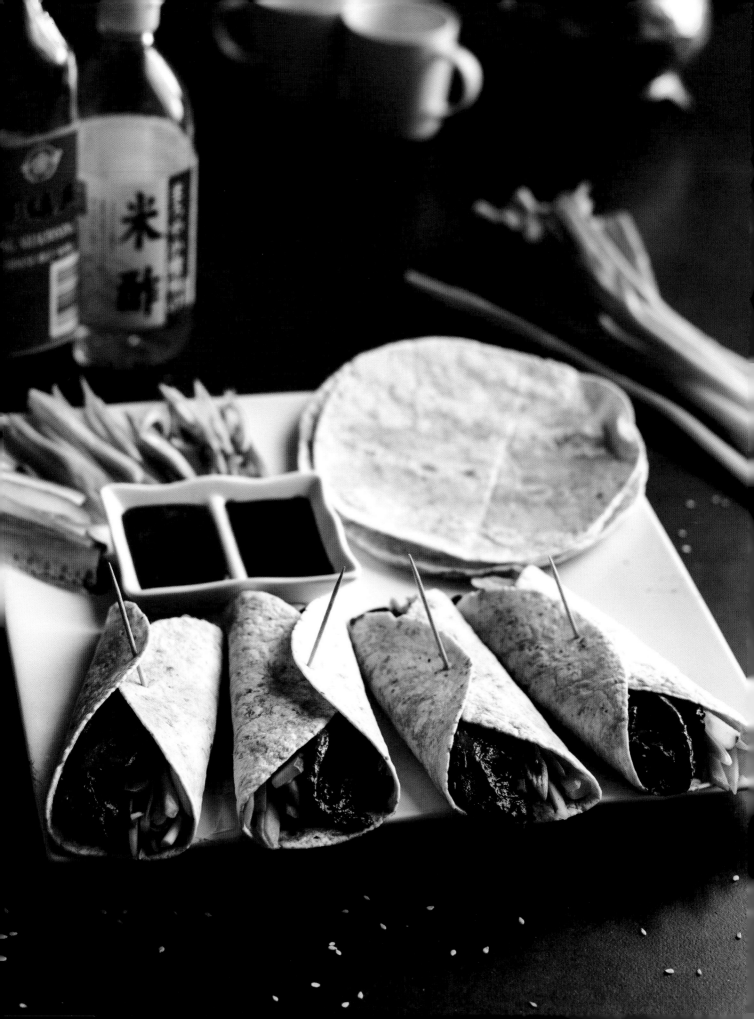

HOISIN MUSHROOM WRAPS

These wraps are so much more exciting than the ubiquitous hummus and avocado ones so often offered as the token vegan option in cafes and supermarkets. Here, sticky hoisin sauce clings to succulent sautéed portobello mushrooms and ginger, which contrasts with crunchy spring onions, carrot and cucumber – all encased in a soft, chewy tortilla wrap to make a sumptuous yet quite light lunch.

Makes: 4 small or 2 large wraps
Equipment: large frying pan, toothpick (cocktail stick), clear film (plastic wrap) (optional)
Prep time: 10 minutes
Cooking time: 20 minutes

30ml/2 tbsp neutral vegetable oil

450g/1lb portobello mushrooms, wiped clean and sliced into thick strips

1cm/½in piece of fresh root ginger, thinly sliced

60ml/4 tbsp hoisin sauce

30ml/2 tbsp rice or white wine vinegar

5ml/1 tsp sesame oil

⅓ large cucumber, sliced into matchsticks

1 small carrot, sliced into matchsticks

2 spring onions (scallions), sliced diagonally

4 small or 2 large tortilla wraps

1 Heat the oil in a large frying pan over a medium-high heat. Add the mushrooms and cook for 15 minutes, adding the ginger after 10 minutes, stirring occasionally. The water from the mushrooms should evaporate and they should shrink.

2 Stir in the hoisin sauce and vinegar and cook for 5 more minutes, then remove from the heat, stir in the sesame oil and leave to cool.

3 If you are making 4 small wraps, arrange one-quarter of the mushroom mixture, cucumber, carrot and spring onions in a line on each wrap. Fold and gently pierce with a toothpick to hold together.

4 If you are using 2 large tortilla wraps, arrange half the mushroom mixture, cucumber, carrot and spring onions in a line, just off centre, on each wrap. Leave about a 2.5cm/1in space at the top and bottom of the wrap. Folding in each end, lift the near edge of the wrap over the filling, then pull towards you to tighten. Tightly roll the wrapped filling to close the wrap. Slice the two wraps in half at a slight angle.

5 If preparing the wraps in advance, wrap tightly in clear film and store in the fridge. They're just as good cold and are great for an office lunch.

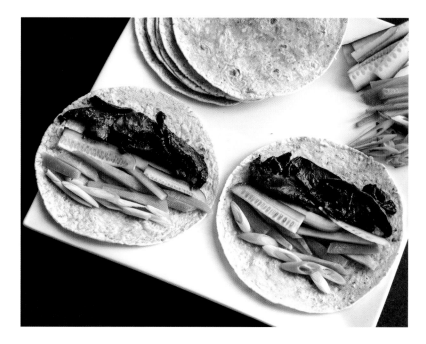

MEXICAN WALNUT BEAN WRAPS

To me, a good wrap is filling but light, and has varying textures and different flavours in each bite –which is absolutely the case here. Walnuts blitzed with earthy spices and paprika make an intriguing Mexican mince-like filling and bring textural contrast to the refried beans and avocado. I like to add few pickled jalapeños for an occasional tangy burst of heat.

Makes: 2 large wraps
Equipment: large frying pan, food processor or blender, clear film (plastic wrap) (optional)
Prep time: 10 minutes
Cooking time: 5 minutes

200g/8oz/2 cups shelled walnuts
67.5ml/4½ tbsp extra virgin olive oil
22.5ml/1½ tbsp soy sauce
3.75ml/¾ tsp ground cumin
3.75ml/¾ tsp ground coriander
3.75ml/¾ tsp smoked paprika
a pinch of cayenne pepper
2 large tortilla wraps
200g/7oz can black beans, drained, rinsed and patted dry
½ ripe avocado, scooped out and chopped
¼ small red onion, finely chopped
6 slices pickled jalapeños (optional)
2 romaine or cos lettuce leaves

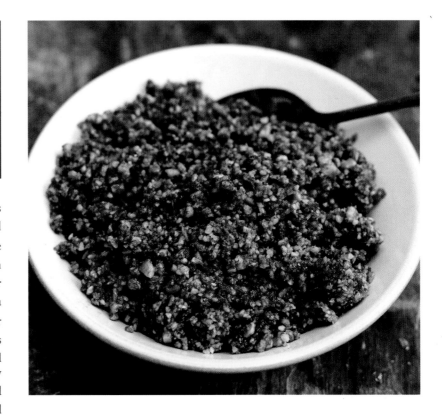

1 Dry-fry the walnuts in a large frying pan over a high heat for 5 minutes, tossing every minute or so, until they are toasted and aromatic. Leave to cool slightly.

2 Put the toasted walnuts, olive oil, soy sauce, cumin, coriander, paprika and cayenne pepper in a food processor or blender and pulse until it has a consistency like minced (ground) meat.

3 Spread out the wraps and arrange half the walnut 'mince', black beans, avocado, red onion, jalapeños and a lettuce leaf in a line, just off centre, on each. Leave about a 2.5cm/1in space at the top and bottom of the wraps.

4 Rotate the wraps so that the line of filling is horizontal to you. Folding in each end, lift the near edge of the wrap over the filling then pull towards you to tighten. Tightly roll the wrapped filling forwards and away from you to close the wrap. Slice the two wraps in half at a slight angle.

5 If preparing for later, wrap tightly in clear film and store in the fridge.

SUBSTITUTE INGREDIENTS
Soy sauce: *tamari sauce*
Cayenne pepper: *chilli powder*
Red onion: *spring onions (scallions)*

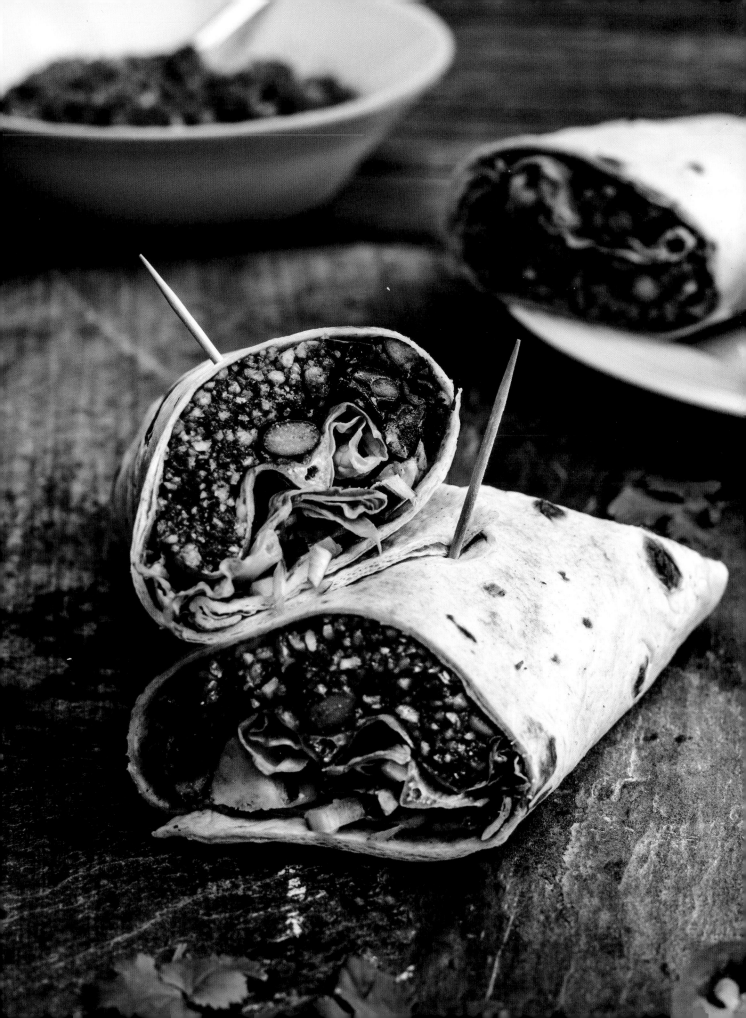

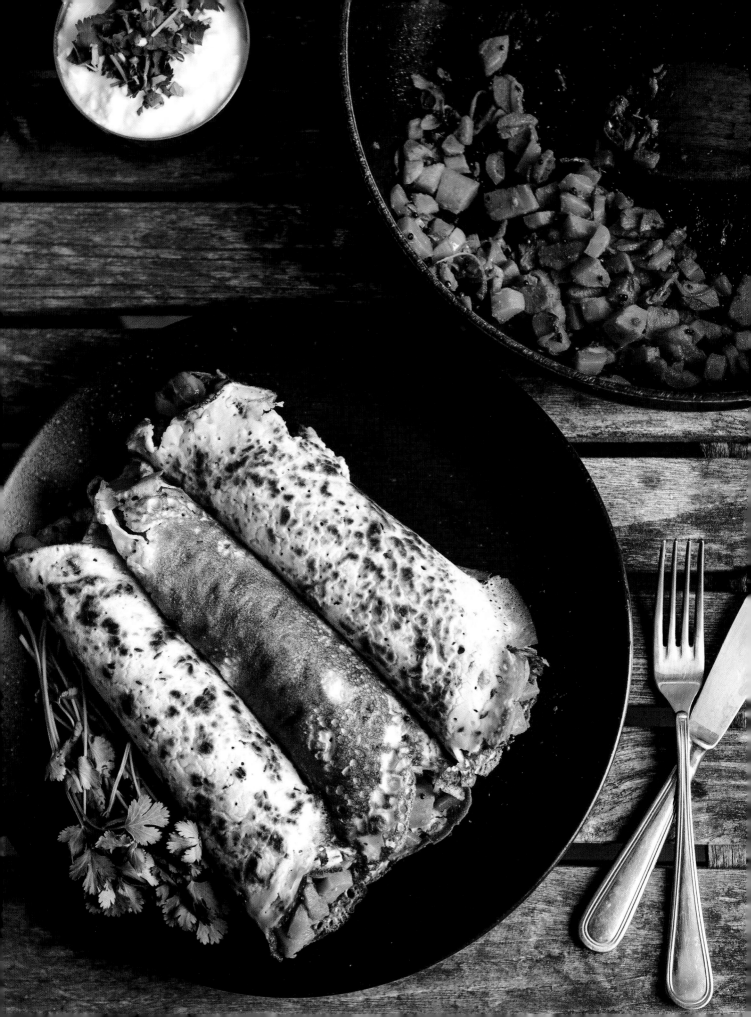

INDIAN FILLED PANCAKES

These are a delicious, aromatic alternative to ordinary savoury pancakes. I particularly like the carrots, the subtle sweetness of which provides welcome contrast to the other, mostly savoury, ingredients. Gram flour adds extra protein and a nice, nutty flavour. Use a good, non-stick frying pan, but regardless, flipping is always a challenge – good luck!

Makes: 4 pancakes (serves 2 generously)
Equipment: medium frying pan, large bowl, medium pan, colander, sieve (strainer), large bowl, whisk, non-stick, wide frying pan, spatula, clean dish towel
Prep time: 20 minutes, plus 10 minutes resting
Cooking time: about 35 minutes

For the pancakes:
10ml/2 tsp cumin seeds
20ml/4 tsp neutral vegetable oil
1 small fresh green chilli, seeded and finely chopped
2 large garlic cloves, finely chopped
2.5cm/1in piece of fresh root ginger, finely chopped
75g/3oz/$\frac{2}{3}$ cup plain (all-purpose) flour
75g/3oz/$\frac{2}{3}$ cup gram (chickpea) flour
2.5ml/$\frac{1}{2}$ tsp fine salt
0.6ml/$\frac{1}{8}$ tsp ground black pepper
350ml/12fl oz/1$\frac{1}{2}$ cups sweetened hemp or other plant-based milk

For the filling:
500g/1$\frac{1}{4}$lb carrots, peeled and diced
20ml/4 tsp neutral vegetable oil
5ml/1 tsp black mustard seeds
1 medium onion, finely sliced
5ml/1 tsp ground turmeric
a pinch of fine salt

To serve (optional):
mango chutney, vegan yogurt and fresh coriander (cilantro)

1 Dry-toast the cumin seeds for the pancakes in a medium frying pan over a medium-high heat for 1–2 minutes, until aromatic. Add 10ml/2 tsp of the oil along with the chilli, garlic and ginger. Fry for 2 minutes, then transfer the mixture to a large bowl and set aside. Don't wash up the frying pan – it will be used again.

2 For the filling, put the carrots in a medium pan, cover with boiling water and cook for 5 minutes, until just soft. Drain in a colander and rinse with cold water to stop them cooking further.

3 In the frying pan, heat the oil over a medium-high heat. Add the mustard seeds and fry for 1–2 minutes. When they start to pop, add the onion and fry for 3 minutes. Stir in the turmeric.

4 Add the boiled and drained carrots to the frying pan and fry for a few minutes, stirring. Remove from the heat and set aside.

5 Sift the plain and chickpea flours for the pancakes into the bowl containing the spice mixture. Add salt and ground black pepper.

6 Pour 120ml/4fl oz/$\frac{1}{2}$ cup of the hemp milk into the bowl, and gently whisk it into the flour. Pour in another 120ml/4fl oz/$\frac{1}{2}$ cup and whisk again, followed by the last of the milk, until you have a smooth, runny consistency. Leave the batter to rest for 10 minutes.

7 In a good non-stick, wide frying pan, heat 2.5ml/$\frac{1}{2}$ tsp of the remaining oil over a medium-high heat. Pour in 100ml/3$\frac{1}{2}$fl oz/scant $\frac{1}{2}$ cup of the batter and tilt the pan so it spreads out. Cook the pancake for 90 seconds–2 minutes. It should be golden brown and crisp.

8 Flip the pancake and cook for a further minute. Transfer to a warm plate and cover to keep warm. Cook the remaining pancakes (there should be enough for 3 more), adding 2.5ml/$\frac{1}{2}$ tsp more oil to the pan each time.

9 When all the pancakes are cooked, place a serving spoonful of the carrots in a line to one side of each pancake. Roll each pancake around the line of carrots and serve, with dollops of mango chutney and vegan yogurt on the side and garnished with fresh coriander, if you like.

RED LENTIL & YELLOW SPLIT PEA DAL

There's no correct English spelling for this dish – dal, daal, dhal, dahl – but one thing is for sure: nearly everyone loves the stuff. Lentils and split peas are filling, healthy and high in protein but also, simmered and cooked into a dal, become unbelievably tasty. I like my dal quite soupy so I can scoop it with a roti instead of using a fork. Leave out some or all of the water at the end for a more fork-ready meal.

Serves: 6
Equipment: strainer, 2 large pans, spoon
Prep time: 15 minutes
Cooking time: 1 hour

225g/8oz/1 cup yellow split peas, rinsed under cold running water
225g/8oz/1 heaped cup dried red lentils
60ml/4 tbsp coconut oil
5ml/1 tsp black mustard seeds
5ml/1 tsp cumin seeds
2 medium onions, finely chopped
4 large garlic cloves, finely chopped
2.5cm/1in piece of fresh root ginger, finely chopped
12.5ml/2½ tsp ground coriander
10ml/2 tsp ground turmeric
1.25ml/¼ tsp chilli powder
1 large tomato, chopped
400g/14oz can light coconut milk or 120ml/4fl oz/½ cup full-fat coconut milk plus 250ml/8fl oz/1 cup water
2.5ml/½ tsp garam masala
10ml/2 tsp fine salt
60ml/4 tbsp finely chopped fresh coriander (cilantro), to garnish
Perfect Basmati Rice (see page 61), naan, roti, or poppadums, to serve

1 Tip the rinsed split peas into one of the large pans and cover with 2 litres/3½ pints/8 cups water. Bring to a boil, skim off any scum or froth with a spoon, then reduce the heat and simmer for 30 minutes.

2 Rinse the red lentils in the strainer, then add to the pan, bring back to a boil, then reduce down to a simmer and continue cooking for another 30 minutes. By the end of the cooking time you should be able to crush a yellow split pea against the side of the pan easily with the back of a spoon.

3 While the lentils are cooking, heat the coconut oil in the other large pan over a medium-high heat. Once the oil is quite hot, add the black mustard and cumin seeds. Fry for 40–60 seconds or until the black mustard seeds start to pop.

4 Lower the heat to medium. Add the onion and cook for 5 minutes, then add the garlic and ginger and cook for a further 10 minutes.

5 Stir in the ground coriander, turmeric, cumin and chilli powder. Cook for 5 more minutes.

6 Add the tomato, turn the heat to low, and gently fry for 10 minutes. Set aside until the lentils have finished cooking.

7 Once the lentils are done, strain them and mix thoroughly into the spiced-onion-tomato mixture.

8 Add the coconut milk and, if you prefer a looser, more soupy dal, a little water. Bring back to a boil, stirring.

9 Remove from the heat, stir in the garam masala and salt, then garnish with the fresh coriander. Serve with basmati rice, naan, roti, or poppadums, if you like.

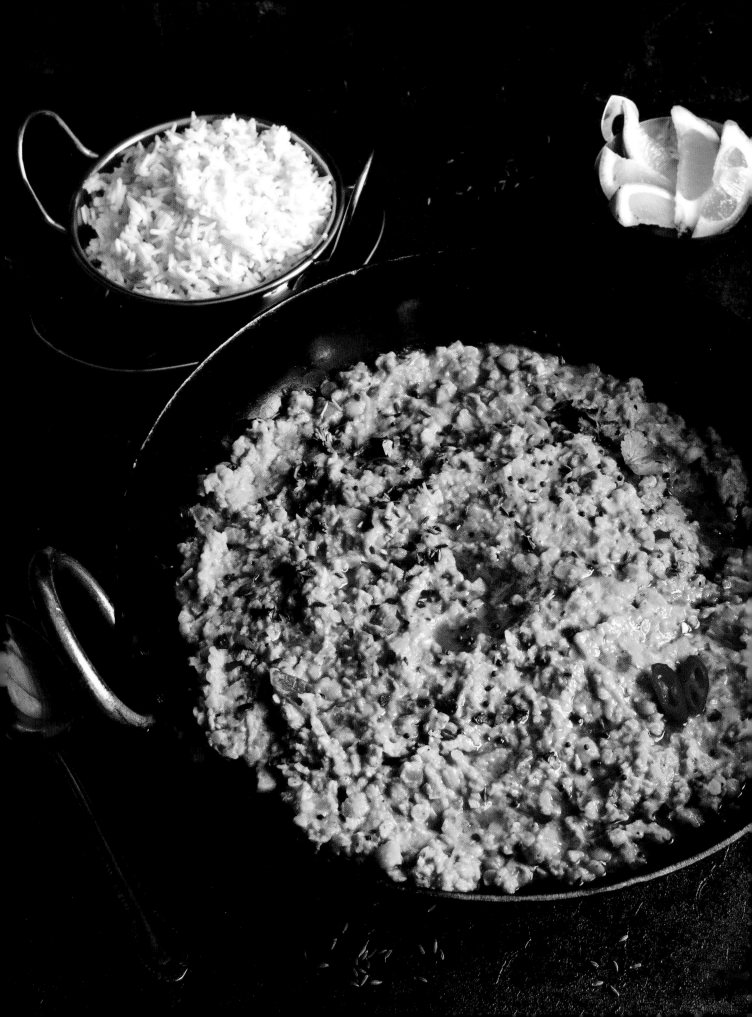

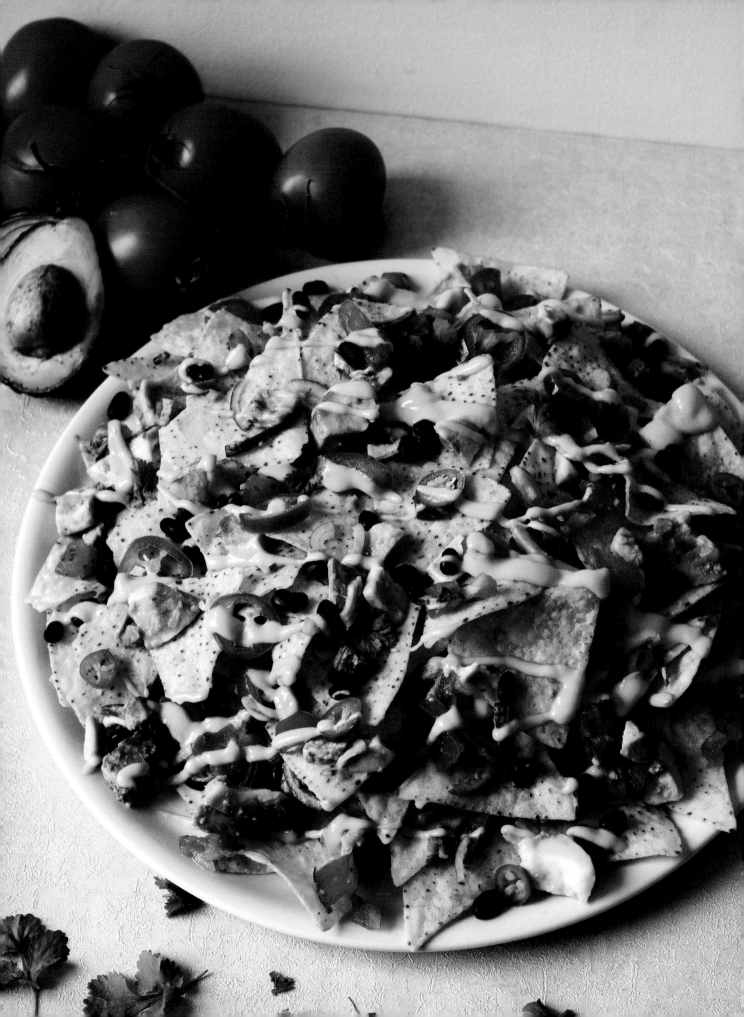

FULLY LOADED NACHOS

Food with layers is more interesting to eat, as every bite catches a little of everything, or gets a bit nearer to the next, more exciting layer. This is very much the case with these nachos, which I've made and devoured too many times to count.

Serves: 4
Equipment: large pan, colander, bowl, strainer, blender or food processor, bowl or jug (pitcher), 2 small bowls, large plate
Prep time: 15 minutes, plus 20 minutes draining
Cooking time: 20 minutes

For the nacho 'cheese' sauce:
200g/7oz floury potatoes, peeled and roughly chopped
1 large carrot, peeled and roughly chopped
2.5ml/½ tsp fine salt
7.5ml/1½ tsp lemon juice
25g/1oz/½ cup nutritional yeast
2.5ml/½ tsp garlic granules or garlic powder
2.5ml/½ tsp onion granules, dried onions or onion powder
90ml/6 tbsp neutral vegetable oil

For the salsa:
300g/11oz ripe tomatoes, chopped
1.25ml/¼ tsp fine salt
¼ medium red onion, chopped
30ml/2 tbsp finely chopped fresh coriander (cilantro)
15ml/1 tbsp lime juice

For the guacamole:
2 medium avocados, scooped out and diced
¼ medium red onion, chopped
0.6ml/⅛ tsp fine salt
15ml/1 tbsp lime juice

To assemble:
400g/14oz tortilla chips, preferably maize
12 pickled jalapeño slices (optional)
200g/7oz can black beans, drained

1 To make the nacho 'cheese' sauce, boil the potatoes and carrot in a large pan with 1 litre/1¾ pints/4 cups water for 15 minutes, until soft. Drain in a colander and rinse with cold water to halt the cooking. Drain well, then transfer to a bowl and set aside.

2 Meanwhile, put the tomatoes for the salsa in a strainer set over the sink and sprinkle with the salt. Leave to drain for 20 minutes.

3 Put all the nacho 'cheese' sauce ingredients apart from the oil, including the potatoes and carrots, in a jug blender or food processor. You could also put them in a bowl and use a stick blender, though the results may not be as smooth.

4 Drizzle the oil in slowly with the motor running, or add it 15ml/1 tbsp at a time if using a stick blender, blitzing in between, until the sauce is thick and smooth. Transfer to a bowl or jug and cover to stop the surface drying out.

5 For the salsa, gently press the last of the juices from the tomatoes, then combine with the onion, coriander and lime juice in a small bowl.

6 For the guacamole, mix the avocado with the onion and salt in another small bowl. Drizzle over the lime juice to prevent the surface from browning, but only gently mix it in properly at the last minute when you are ready to eat.

7 On a large plate or platter, spread out one-third of the tortilla chips as a base layer. Sprinkle over one-third of the guacamole, one-third of the salsa and one-third of the nacho 'cheese' sauce. Add a few jalapeño slices, if using, and some black beans.

8 Add another one-third of the tortilla chips on top, then repeat the previous step two more times, drizzling extra cheese sauce over the top. Serve immediately.

SAUSAGE ROLL BITES

Who would have thought sausage rolls would be so easy to make, and be vegan at that? The store-bought ones seem artificial and manufactured, as if such a thing can only be made by machine. However, some ready-made puff pastry is already vegan and meat-free minces are excellent now, so all you need do is a little sautéing, rolling and slicing, and then give them a quick blast in the oven! Easy as ... vegan sausage rolls!

Makes: 12 sausage rolls
Equipment: large baking tray, baking parchment, medium frying pan, large bowl, knife, rolling pin, pastry brush, small bowl, wire rack
Prep time: 25 minutes
Cooking time: 40 minutes

45ml/3 tbsp olive oil
1 medium red or white onion, finely chopped
2 sage leaves, chopped
350g/12oz frozen vegan meat-free mince*
60ml/4 tbsp dried or fresh breadcrumbs
2.5ml/½ tsp ground white pepper
2.5ml/½ tsp fine salt
500g/1¼lb ready-made vegan puff pastry
flour, for dusting
10ml/2 tsp soya milk

For the glaze:
10ml/2 tsp soya milk
5ml/1 tsp maple syrup

* The best types of vegan 'mince' are made of rehydrated textured vegetable protein, aka soya. Some mainstream supermarkets make an own-brand version that is vegan – usually frozen not fresh.

1 Preheat the oven to 180°C/350°F/Gas 4. Line a large baking tray with baking parchment.

2 Heat the oil in a medium frying pan over a medium heat. Add the onion and sage and sauté for 5 minutes. Add the meat-free mince and cook for 10 more minutes, stirring frequently, until evenly cooked.

3 Transfer this mixture to a large bowl along with the breadcrumbs, white pepper and salt. Add 30ml/2 tbsp water and mix well.

4 Cut the pastry block into two equal rectangles. Sprinkle a little flour on a kitchen work surface. Flour your rolling pin and roll each pastry rectangle out to approximately 40 x 30cm/16 x 12in each.

5 Arrange half the sausage mixture along each pastry rectangle, lengthways, leaving a 2.5cm/1in edge on one side. Gently press the filling mixture together into a neater, firmer line.

6 Brush the long edges of the pastry with the soya milk using a pastry brush, then roll it firmly from the side nearest the filling to form a long cylinder, pressing down to seal. Repeat with the other pastry rectangle. Cut each pastry cylinder into 6 pieces and transfer to the lined baking tray.

7 Mix the soya milk and maple syrup in a small bowl, then brush the glaze all over the pastry. Bake for 25 minutes. Remove from the oven, transfer to a wire rack and leave to cool slightly before devouring.

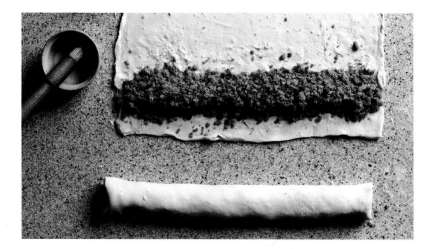

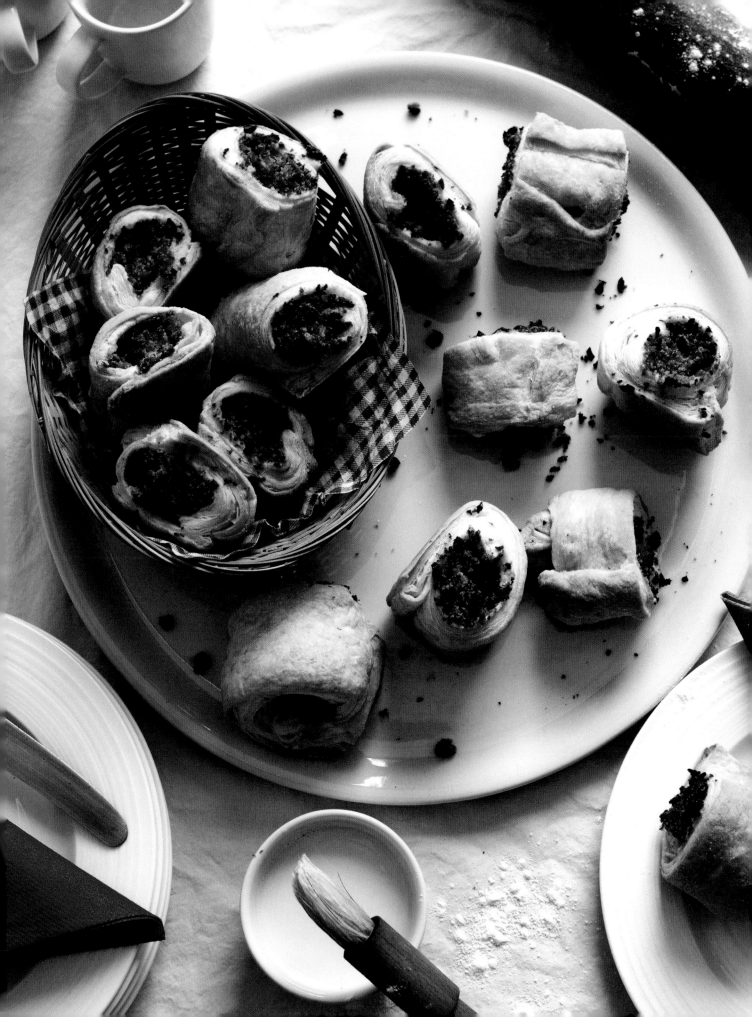

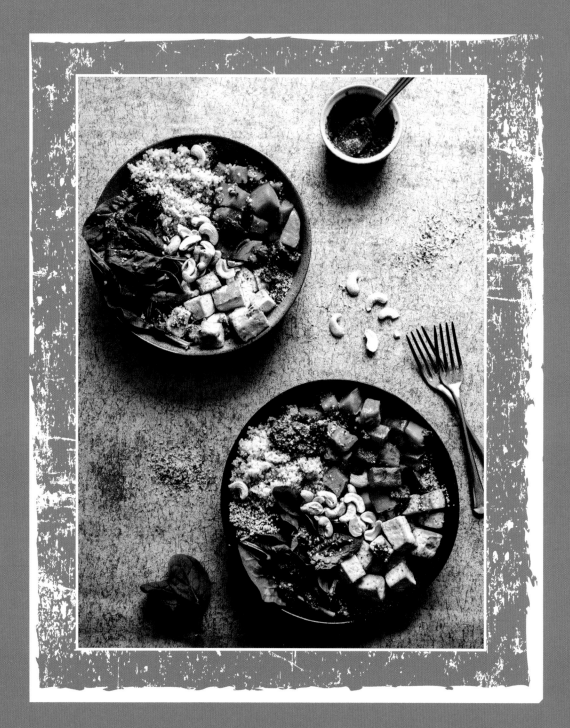

SOUPS AND SALADS

MISO SOUP WITH CAVOLO NERO

Serves: 4
Equipment: cloth or kitchen paper, large pan or casserole
Prep time: 5 minutes
Cooking time: 15 minutes

Miso soup can appear sophisticated but it's actually super simple to make. Miso paste is a fermented soy product, so has a beneficial effect on your gut health. You can find kombu (a type of Japanese seaweed) in Asian supermarkets – it's one of the two components of a classic dashi stock, and it adds a nice, umami flavour – but it isn't essential. I like to add cavolo nero to the soup for a fresh, earthy nutrition boost.

10 sq cm/4 sq in piece of kombu (optional)

4 large leaves cavolo nero (about 115g/4oz), roughly chopped

45ml/3 tbsp brown/red miso paste

300g/11oz silken tofu, drained and cubed (optional)

2 spring onions (scallions), thinly sliced crossways

10ml/2 tsp sesame seeds

15ml/1 tbsp toasted sesame oil

1 If using, wipe the kombu with a cloth or piece of kitchen paper to get rid of any dirt, being careful not to wipe away the white powder.

2 Place the kombu in a large pan or casserole with 1 litre/1¾pints/4 cups water. Turn the heat on to medium and bring to a very low simmer (do not bring to a boil). Once at a low simmer, turn the heat down to low. Add the cavolo nero and simmer gently for 10 minutes.

3 Remove and discard the kombu, then add the miso. Bring to a boil, stirring so the miso dissolves. Taste the soup and add more water if it's too strong, or more miso paste if it isn't strong enough.

4 Turn off the heat and add the silken tofu, if using. Serve topped with the spring onions, sesame seeds and toasted sesame oil.

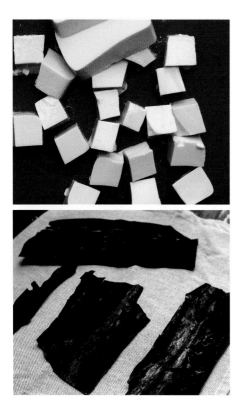

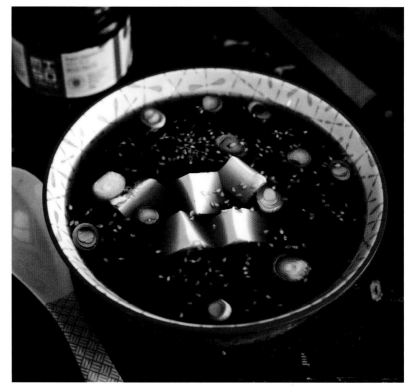

PEA & MINT SOUP

Serves: 4
Equipment: large pan or casserole,
jug blender or stick blender
Prep time: 5 minutes
Cooking time: 25 minutes

60ml/4 tbsp olive oil
1 large leek, whites only, finely chopped
1 small onion, finely chopped
500g/1¼lb/4¼ cups frozen peas
a large handful (about 20) of fresh
mint leaves
60ml/4 tbsp soya cream (optional)
5ml/1 tsp fine salt

To garnish (optional):
a little chopped fresh mint
a splash of soya cream
ground black pepper

I love how pea soup can be a healthy, refreshing dish at the same time as a creamy, almost indulgent, restaurant-style soup – it's the best of both worlds. Be sure to only use frozen peas, which are frozen very quickly after picking and retain all their freshness and vibrancy. Hemp milk is used here as it's quite sweet and creamy. The salt may seem too much, but it's needed to complement the sweetness of the peas.

1 Heat the oil in a large pan or casserole over a medium-low heat. Add the leek and onion and sauté for 15 minutes.

2 Add the peas, mint and 750ml/1¼ pints/3 cups water and bring to a boil. Turn down to a simmer, cover and cook for 10 minutes.

3 Add the soya cream (if using), then transfer everything to a jug blender and blitz to a smooth, creamy soup. This could also be done with a stick blender in the pan, but it will take longer to achieve a smooth consistency.

4 Stir in the salt, then ladle into bowls and garnish with chopped mint, a splash of soya cream and a good grind of black pepper.

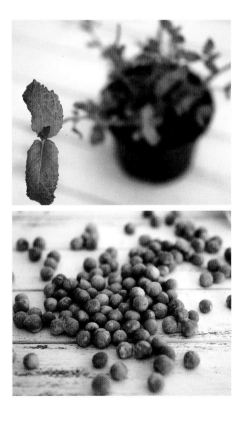
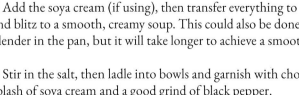

HEARTY WINTER VEGETABLE SOUP

Monday. January. Wake up cold. Get colder on way to work. Office heating broken. Fingers numb. Feet may have fallen off. Shivering by 5. Home, cold to your bones. Nothing but a hot bath and a bowl of this soup will do for you now. Restored. Repeat.

Serves: 4
Equipment: large pan or casserole, jug blender or stick blender
Prep time: 15 minutes
Cooking time: 55 minutes

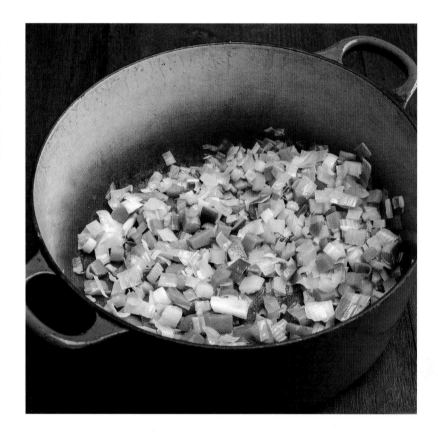

60ml/4 tbsp olive oil
1 large carrot, diced
1 leek, white and green parts, diced
2 celery sticks, diced
3 sprigs of fresh thyme, leaves only
2 bay leaves
1kg/2¼lb root vegetables, such as swede (rutabaga), celeriac, parsnip and turnip, peeled and chopped
475ml/16fl oz/2 cups unsweetened plant-based milk
5ml/1 tsp fine salt
2.5ml/½ tsp ground black pepper
60ml/4 tbsp soya cream (optional)

To serve (optional):
a splash of soya cream
a pinch of ground black pepper
a sprinkling of pumpkin and sunflower seeds, roasted
thick slices of toast

1 Heat the oil over a medium-high heat in a large pan or casserole. Add the carrot, leek and celery and fry for 5 minutes, stirring occasionally.

2 Add the thyme and bay leaves and cook for 5 more minutes, then add the root vegetables, plant-based milk and 1 litre/1¾ pints/4 cups water. Bring to a boil, then turn the heat down to a simmer, cover and cook for about 45 minutes, until the vegetables are really soft.

3 Stir in the salt and ground black pepper and add the soya cream, if using.

4 Remove the bay leaves, then transfer everything to a jug blender and blitz to a smooth, creamy soup. This could also be done with a stick blender in the pan if you like, though it will take longer to achieve a smooth consistency. Add a splash of water if the soup is too thick.

5 Serve topped with a splash of soya cream, a good pinch of ground black pepper and a few pumpkin and sunflower seeds, and with some thick toast for dunking alongside, if you like.

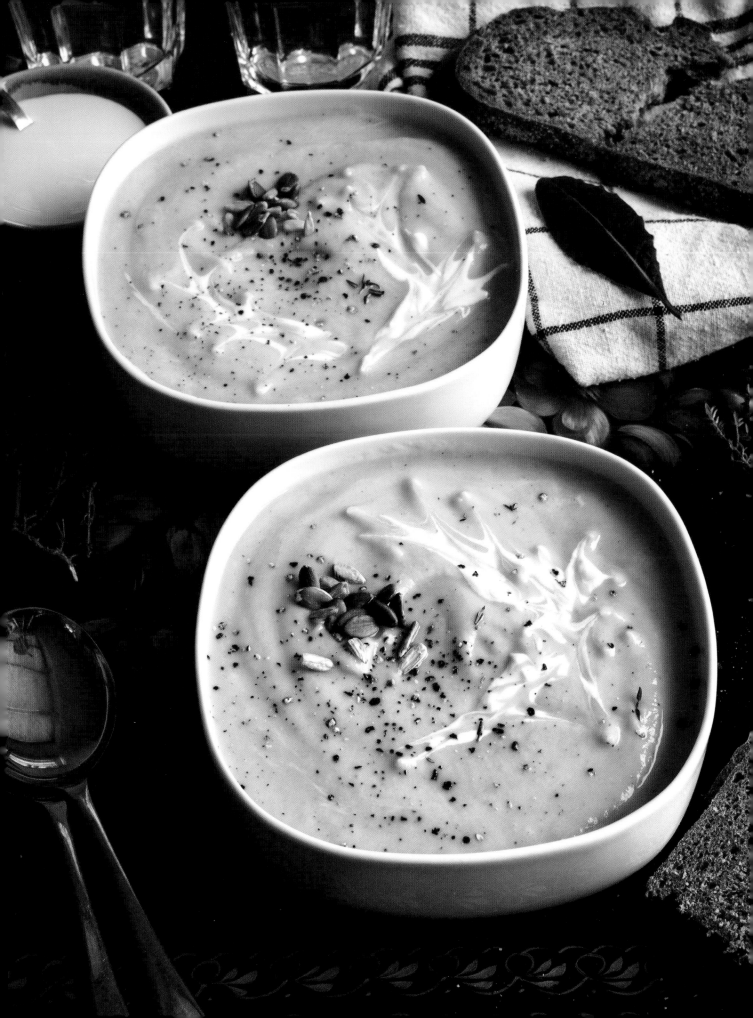

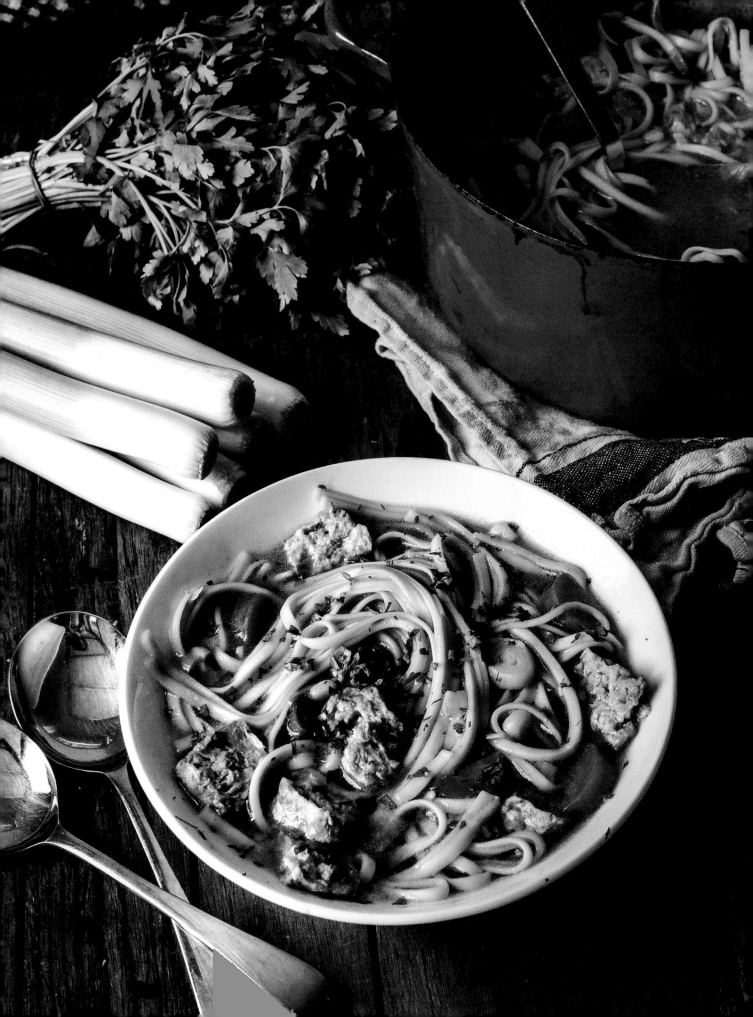

'CHICKEN' NOODLE SOUP

Eat this when you're ill. And eat it when you're not ill. Nowadays, substitute chicken pieces are very good and, especially in a soup like this, will taste near indistinguishable from real chicken – if that's what you crave.

Serves: 4
Equipment: large pan or casserole, strainer, large bowl
Prep time: 30 minutes
Cooking time: about 1 hour 25 minutes

For the stock:
60ml/4 tbsp neutral vegetable oil
115g/4oz button (white) mushrooms, halved
1 medium onion, roughly chopped
1 medium carrot, roughly chopped
1 celery stick, roughly chopped
4 whole black peppercorns
2 garlic cloves, peeled and sliced
1 fresh or dried bay leaf
2 sprigs of fresh thyme
10 medium dried porcini mushroom pieces
15ml/1 tbsp soy sauce

For the soup:
1 large leek, chopped
1 large carrot, diced
300g/11oz vegan chicken pieces, e.g. Quorn/Gardein
200g/7oz udon (wheat) noodles
200g/7oz can corn, drained
salt or soy sauce, and ground black pepper
30ml/2 tbsp finely chopped parsley

SUBSTITUTE INGREDIENTS
Button mushrooms: *chestnut mushrooms*
Soy sauce: *tamari sauce*
Udon noodles: *rice or buckwheat noodles*

1 Heat 30ml/2 tbsp of the oil in a large pan or casserole over a high heat. Add the mushrooms and fry for 10 minutes so they get a good amount of colour. Add 30ml/2 tbsp more oil to the pan along with the onion, carrot, celery and peppercorns. Fry for 5 minutes, still over a high heat.

2 Add the garlic to the pan and fry for 1–2 minutes, then add the bay leaf, thyme, porcini mushrooms and soy sauce along with 1.5 litres/ 2½ pints/6¼ cups water. Bring to a boil, then turn down to a low simmer, cover and leave to cook for 45 minutes.

3 Drain the stock through a strainer into a large bowl. Press the vegetables down to release as much liquid as possible. Discard the vegetable mush. Pour the stock back into the large pan or casserole.

4 Add the leek, carrot and vegan chicken pieces to the stock and bring back to a boil. Reduce the heat to a simmer and cook for the time stated on the chicken pieces' packaging (normally around 15 minutes).

5 Once the carrot, leek and chicken pieces are cooked, add half the chopped parsley and the noodles to the pan, bring to a boil, then reduce the heat and simmer for the time stated on the noodle packaging. Add some water if there isn't enough to easily submerge the noodles.

6 Stir in the corn. Taste and adjust the seasoning with salt or a dash of soy sauce and black pepper. Serve, topped with the remaining parsley.

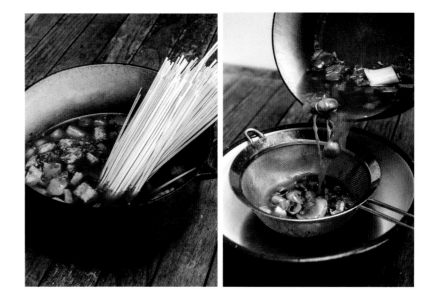

QUICK RAMEN

Versatility, speed and flavour. Tick, tick and tick. I make this for lunch a couple times a week, with leftover tare sauce (a delicious Japanese dipping sauce, see below), and in 10 minutes have a big bowl of steaming-hot noodles in aromatic broth, with crunchy veg piled on top. Heaven.

Serves: 4
Equipment: kitchen paper, plate, small bowl, fork or whisk, wok, tongs or a spatula, large plate or baking tray, dish towel or foil, large pan, colander, kettle
Prep time: 20 minutes
Cooking time: 5–10 minutes

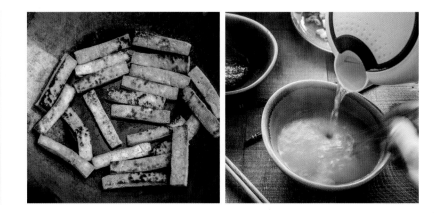

For the tare sauce:
100g/3¾oz/⅓ cup brown/red miso paste

60ml/4 tbsp tahini

60ml/4 tbsp soy or tamari sauce

15ml/1 tbsp vegetable stock concentrate or 1 vegetable stock (bouillon) cube

2.5cm/1in piece of fresh root ginger, grated or 30ml/2 tbsp garlic-ginger paste

1 garlic clove, crushed

22.5ml/1½ tbsp sesame oil

a pinch of chilli powder

For the toppings:
400g/14oz block extra-firm tofu, drained

45ml/3 tbsp neutral vegetable oil

150g/5oz Chinese leaf or white cabbage, sliced into strips

1 large carrot, sliced into strips

3 spring onions (scallions), sliced

20ml/4 tsp black or white sesame seeds

For the noodles:
300g/11oz wheat (udon or ramen), rice or buckwheat noodles

1 Press the water out of the tofu for the topping by placing the block between two layers of kitchen paper on a plate and pressing down firmly with your hands. Slice into strips and set aside.

2 To make the tare sauce, whisk together all of the ingredients in a small bowl using a fork or small whisk.

3 For the toppings, heat 22.5ml/1½ tbsp of the oil over a very high heat in a wok. Fry the tofu strips for around 2 minutes, until crispy and browned on each side, being careful not to break them (use tongs or a spatula to turn them over). Transfer to a large plate or baking tray and cover with a clean dish towel or some foil so the tofu doesn't get cold.

4 Now stir-fry the cabbage and carrot in the remaining vegetable oil in the wok for around 2 minutes. Transfer to the plate or tray containing the tofu.

5 Cook your choice of noodles in a large pan of boiling water according to packet instructions, erring on the side of slightly undercooked. Drain well in a colander.

6 Boil 1.5 litres/2½ pints/6¼ cups water in a kettle. Have four serving bowls ready to fill. Put 30ml/2 tbsp of the tare into each bowl, then pour over boiling water so each bowl is around two-thirds full. Whisk the water into the tare using the fork or whisk. It should make a thick, creamy broth.

7 Divide the noodles between the bowls and top each bowl with tofu, cabbage, carrot, spring onions and sesame seeds. Eat with chopsticks, if you like. Slurping is encouraged.

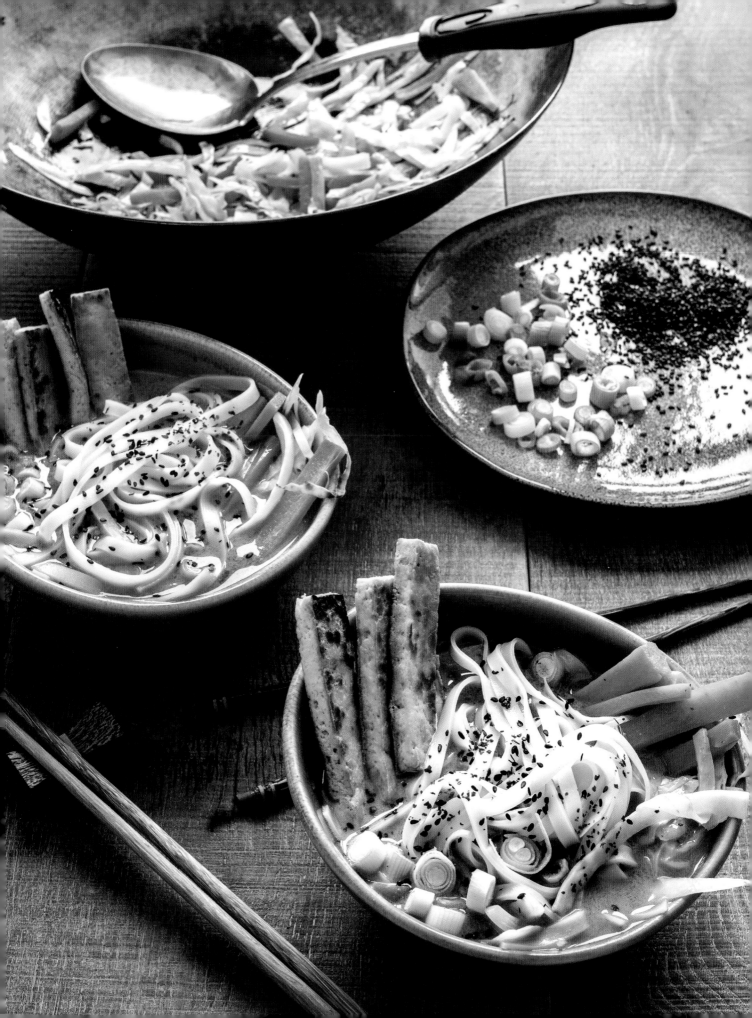

ULTIMATE VEGAN RAMEN

Serves: 6
Equipment: large pan or casserole with a lid, damp cloth (optional), kitchen paper, plate, small bowl, fork or whisk, colander, large bowl, wok, large plate or baking tray, clean dish towel or foil, large pan
Prep time: 40 minutes
Cooking time: about 1 hour 10 minutes

Don't attempt this recipe when you are tired or after a long day of work. Make it instead over a weekend when you have time on your hands, friends to impress or just an ambitious appetite. You will be richly rewarded.

1 First, make the broth. Heat 30ml/2 tbsp of the oil in a large pan over a high heat. Fry the mushrooms for 10 minutes so they get a good amount of colour and any liquid released has disappeared.

2 Add the remaining 15ml/1 tbsp vegetable oil to the pan along with the onion, carrot, spring onions, celery and peppercorns. Fry for 5 minutes, still over a high heat. Add the ginger and garlic to the pan and fry for 1–2 more minutes, then add the porcini mushrooms along with 3 litres/5 pints/12½ cups water.

3 Wipe any dirt off the kombu with a damp cloth or kitchen paper, being careful not to wipe away the white powder. Add it to the broth. Bring to a boil, then reduce to a low simmer, cover and leave to cook for 45 minutes.

4 Meanwhile, press the water out of the tofu for the topping by placing the block between two layers of kitchen paper on a plate and pressing down firmly with your hands. Slice into 2.5cm/1in cubes.

5 For the tare, put all the ingredients in a small bowl and whisk into a thick paste using a fork or whisk. Set aside.

6 Drain the broth through a colander into a large bowl. Press the vegetables down to release as much liquid as possible. Discard all the vegetables, then pour the stock back into the large pan or casserole and add the sesame oil.

7 Now cook the toppings: heat 5ml/1 tsp of the vegetable oil over a very high heat in a wok. Stir-fry the cabbage for 45–60 seconds, then transfer to a large plate and cover to keep warm.

8 Stir-fry the tofu in another 5ml/1 tsp vegetable oil for 90 seconds, until crispy and browned, then transfer to the plate with the cabbage. Stir-fry the mushroom strips in the remaining oil for 90 seconds and transfer to the plate. Add the sesame oil and toss to combine.

9 Place the bean sprouts, corn, spring onions and sesame seeds on another plate so they're to hand for assembly. Cook the ramen noodles in a large pan of boiling water according to packet instructions. Drain and leave in the colander. Bring the stock back to the boil.

10 Warm six large bowls and place on the work surface. Put 30ml/2 tbsp of the tare in the bottom of each bowl, then pour over the broth so each bowl is around two-thirds full. Whisk the broth into the tare.

For the broth:
45ml/3 tbsp neutral vegetable oil
225g/8oz button (white) mushrooms
1 medium onion, roughly chopped
1 medium carrot, roughly chopped
6 spring onions (scallions), sliced
2 celery sticks, roughly chopped
6 whole black peppercorns
2.5cm/1in piece of fresh root ginger, sliced
4 garlic cloves, sliced
15 medium dried porcini mushroom pieces
10 sq cm/4 sq in piece of kombu
15ml/1 tbsp sesame oil

For the tare sauce:
150g/5oz/½ cup brown/red miso paste
60ml/4 tbsp tahini
30ml/2 tbsp sesame oil
4 medium garlic cloves, grated or crushed
2.5cm/1in piece of fresh root ginger, grated
60ml/4 tbsp soy sauce
1.25ml/¼ tsp chilli powder

For the toppings:
400g/14oz block extra-firm tofu, drained
15ml/1 tbsp neutral vegetable oil
100g/3¾ white cabbage, sliced into strips
150g/5oz shiitake or portobello mushrooms, sliced into strips
7.5ml/½ tbsp sesame oil
300g/11oz/3 cups bean sprouts

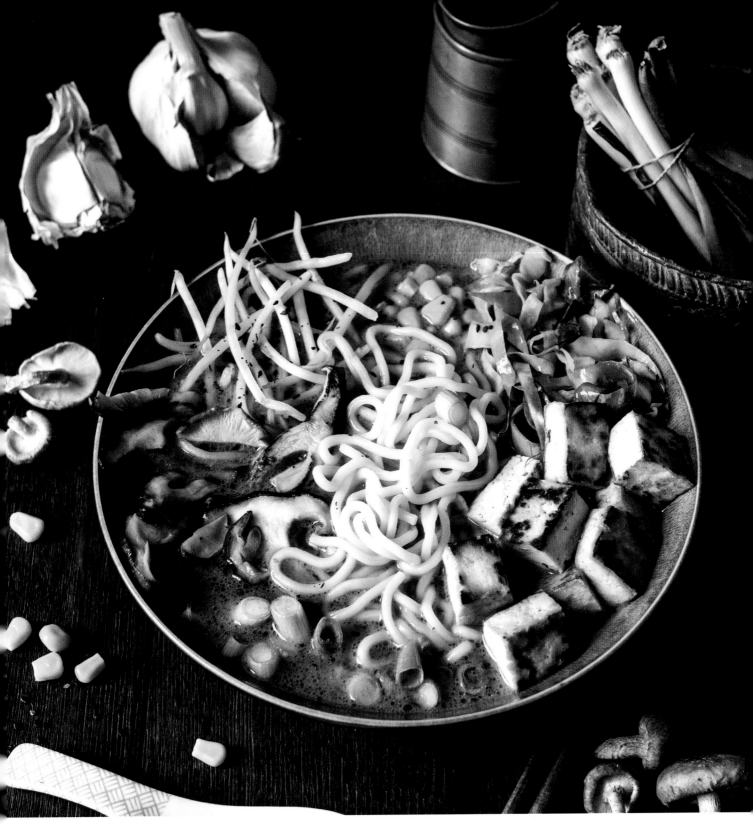

200g/7oz can corn, drained

3 spring onions (scallions), very thinly sliced

30ml/2 tbsp black or white sesame seeds

900g/2lb frozen or vacuum-packed fresh ramen noodles

30ml/2 tbsp chiu chow chilli oil (optional)

11 Add a dash of chilli oil to each bowl (if using), then divide the noodles evenly between the bowls.

12 Top each bowl with cabbage, tofu, mushrooms, bean sprouts, corn, spring onions and a sprinkling of sesame seeds. Eat with chopsticks, if you like.

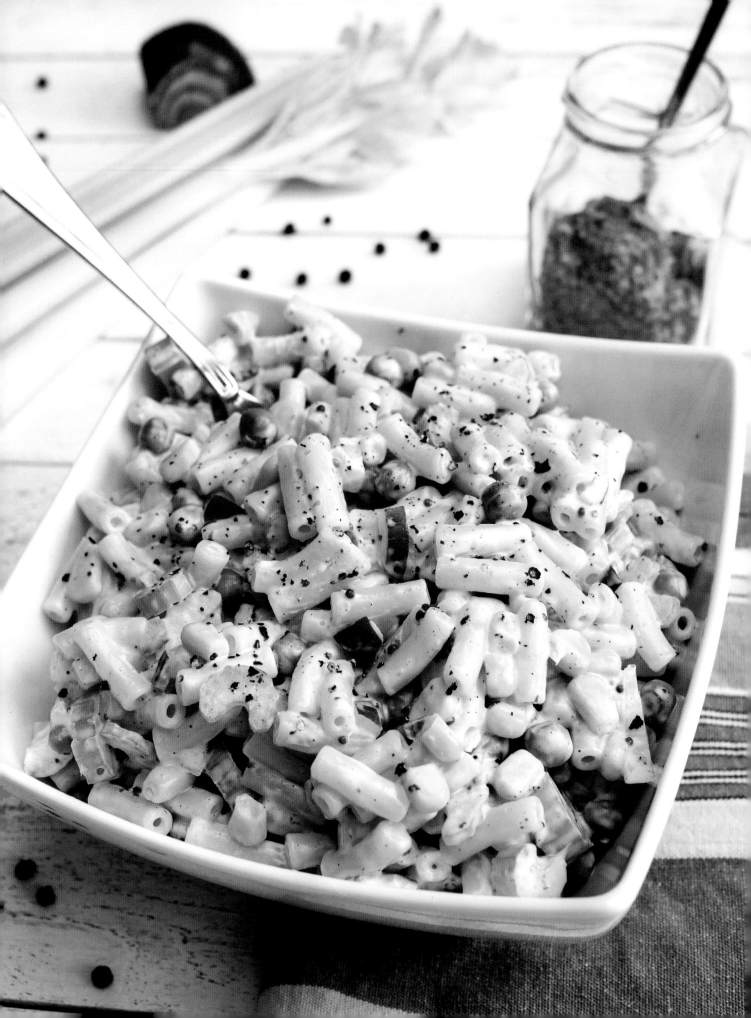

CREAMY PASTA SALAD

Don't let the word 'salad' fool you, here. This dish is instant satisfaction: to tuck in to straight from the fridge or to take to work when you won't have a chance to eat for the next few hours. In my opinion, it's better fridge-cold. Maybe that's just me.

Serves: 4
Equipment: large bowl, large pan, colander,
Prep time: 10 minutes
Cooking time: about 10 minutes

For the dressing:
225g/8oz/1 cup vegan mayonnaise
15ml/1 tbsp wholegrain mustard
15ml/1 tbsp lemon juice
15ml/1 tbsp cider vinegar
5ml/1 tsp onion granules, onion powder
or dried onions
5ml/1 tsp garlic granules or garlic powder
1.25ml/¼ tsp caster (superfine) sugar
2.5ml/½ tsp fine salt
1.25ml/¼ tsp ground black pepper

For the pasta:
7.5ml/1½ tsp fine salt
275g/10oz/3 cups dried elbow macaroni
175g/7oz/1½ cups frozen peas

For the other vegetables:
2 celery sticks, sliced
½ small red onion, chopped
200g/7oz can corn, drained and rinsed

1 Mix all the dressing ingredients thoroughly in a large bowl. Set aside.

2 For the pasta, bring 2 litres/3½ pints/8 cups water to a boil in a large pan. Add the salt and boil the pasta until al dente, according to the packet instructions, adding the peas for the final 3 minutes.

3 Drain the pasta and peas in a colander and rinse thoroughly with cold water to stop them cooking further. Shake the colander to drain off as much excess water as possible.

4 Add the pasta and peas to the dressing, along with the celery, red onion and corn, and stir well to combine.

5 Eat immediately, or store in an airtight container and chill first for a couple of hours and then eat straight from the fridge. You can eat this the next day, it keeps really well, and it's also a great picnic dish.

SUBSTITUTE INGREDIENTS
Wholegrain mustard: *Dijon mustard*
Onion granules: *nutritional yeast*
Macaroni: *fusilli, penne, conchiglie*

POWER BOWL I

This bowl contains a hefty whack of plant-based protein and plenty of unsaturated fats and complex carbohydrates. Oh, and vitamins and minerals to boot! Idea: cook double the quantity of spelt, edamame and black beans, store in containers in the fridge, and you can put together a bowl in 5 minutes. Now that's power.

Makes: 2–3 bowls
Equipment: strainer, large pan, small bowl, fork, microwave-safe bowl (optional)
Prep time: 15 minutes
Cooking time: 20 minutes

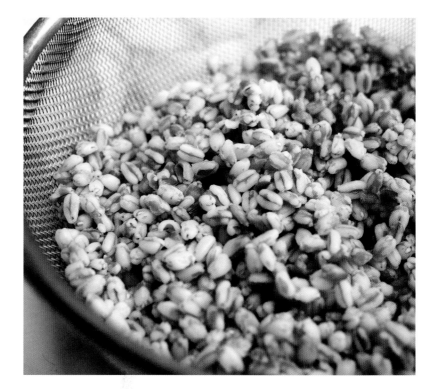

100g/3¾oz/½ cup spelt
1.25ml/¼ tsp fine salt
150g/5oz/1 cup frozen edamame beans
400g/14oz can black beans, drained and rinsed
½ avocado, flesh sliced
60g/2½oz/2 packed handfuls of baby spinach leaves
45ml/3 tbsp pumpkin seeds
45ml/3 tbsp almonds, roughly chopped
15ml/1 tbsp chia seeds

For the dressing:
45ml/3 tbsp tahini
10ml/2 tsp soy sauce
5ml/1 tsp maple syrup
5ml/1 tsp rice or white wine vinegar

SUBSTITUTE INGREDIENTS
Spelt: *brown rice, bulgur wheat or faro, cooked*
Black beans: *cannellini or borlotti beans*
Pumpkin seeds: *sunflower seeds*
Almonds: *macadamia or cashew nuts*
Chia seeds: *sesame or hemp seeds*
Tahini: *almond or peanut butter*

1 Put the spelt in a strainer, rinse well and transfer to a large pan. Add 750ml/1¼ pints/3 cups water and the salt, bring to a boil, turn the heat down to a simmer and cook for 20 minutes. Drain well.

2 Meanwhile, make the dressing. In a small bowl, whisk together all the ingredients using a fork. Stir in water to loosen to a pourable consistency. Set aside.

3 Cook the edamame beans by microwaving for 4 minutes in a microwave-safe bowl. Alternatively, add them to the simmering spelt for the final 4 minutes of the cooking time.

4 To assemble, place some cooked spelt, edamame beans, black beans, avocado and spinach leaves next to each other in wide bowls.

5 Sprinkle the pumpkin seeds, almonds and chia seeds over the top, then drizzle over the dressing and serve. Alternatively, leave out the avocado and pack the rest into airtight containers to store in the fridge until required, then add the avocado at the last minute.

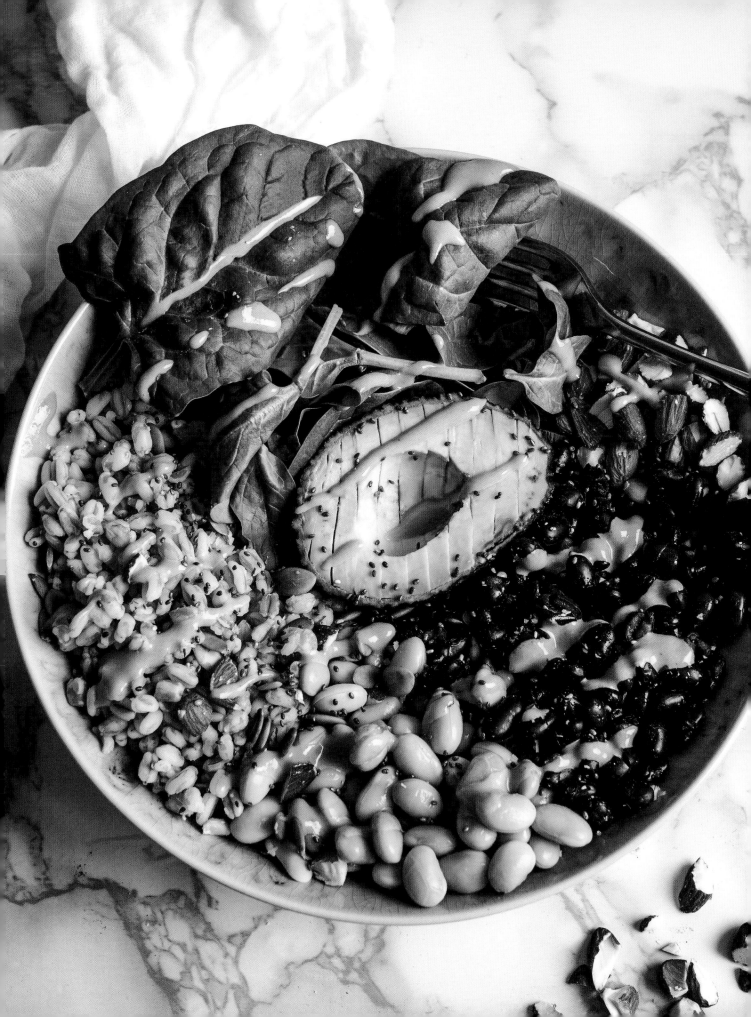

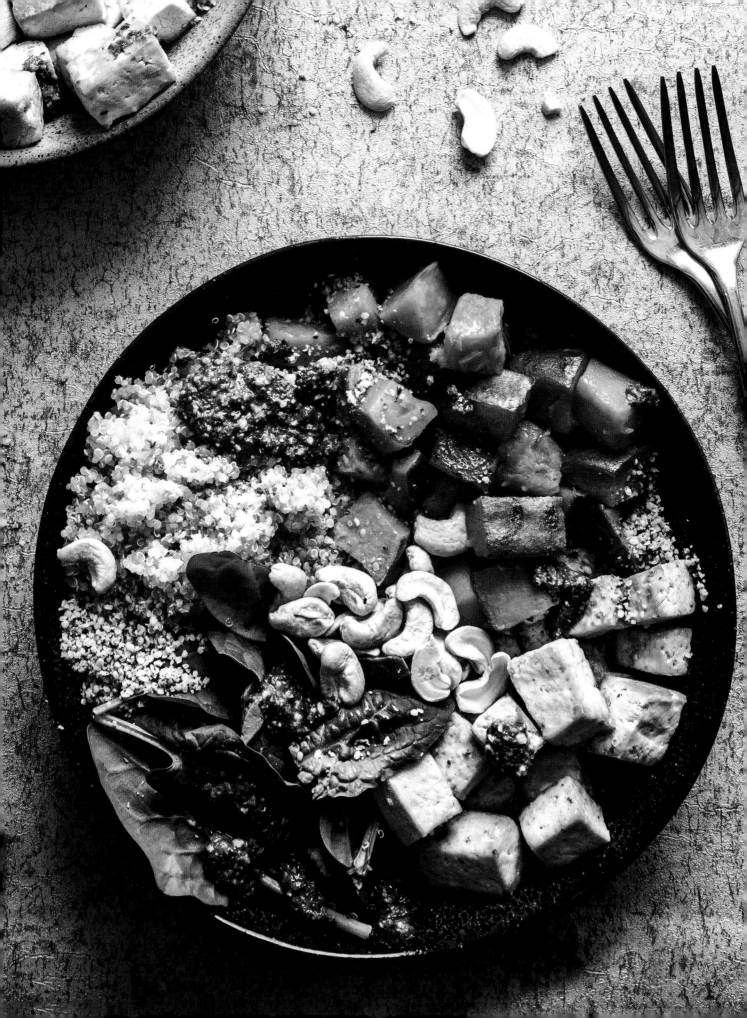

POWER BOWL II

This power-packed super-bowl is also rammed with protein, complex carbs, vitamins, minerals and good fats. As with the other power bowl, you could double (or even triple) the tofu, sweet potato and quinoa, store in containers in the fridge, and make lunch for the next few days in minutes. If you have a smaller appetite, the quantities given may be enough for three people/bowls.

Makes: 2–3 bowls
Equipment: kitchen paper, plate, small baking tray, strainer, large pan, wide serving bowls
Prep time: 15 minutes
Cooking time: 20 minutes

400g/14oz block extra-firm tofu, drained
1 medium sweet potato, cubed
30ml/2 tbsp olive oil
2.5ml/½ tsp fine salt
75g/3oz/½ cup quinoa
45ml/3 tbsp Versatile Vegan Pesto (see page 32) or store-bought vegan pesto
50g/2oz/2 packed handfuls of baby spinach leaves
30ml/2 tbsp hemp seeds
50g/2oz/⅓ cup cashew nuts

1 Preheat the oven to 180°C/350°F/Gas 4.

2 Press the water out of the tofu by placing the block of tofu between two layers of kitchen paper on a plate and pressing down firmly with your hands. Slice into 2.5cm/1in cubes.

3 Once the oven is hot, put the pressed tofu and sweet potato on a small baking tray and toss with the olive oil and 1.25ml/¼ tsp of the salt. Roast in the oven for 20 minutes.

4 Meanwhile, put the quinoa in a strainer, rinse well and transfer to a large pan. Add 400ml/14fl oz/1⅔ cups water and the remaining salt, bring to a boil, turn the heat down to a simmer and cook for about 15 minutes, until all the water is absorbed.

5 While the tofu, sweet potato and quinoa are cooking, stir 15–30ml/1–2 tbsp water into the pesto so you have a pourable dressing.

6 To assemble, place some tofu, sweet potato, quinoa and spinach leaves snugly next to each other in wide bowls. Sprinkle the hemp seeds and cashews over the top, then drizzle over the dressing and serve, or pack into airtight containers and store in the fridge, as required.

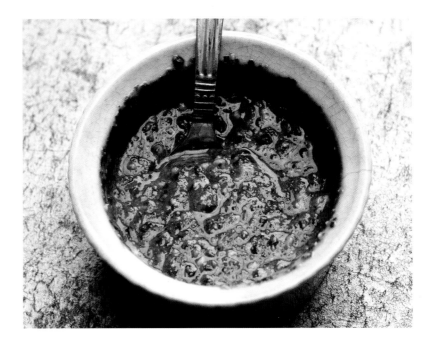

> **SUBSTITUTE INGREDIENTS**
> Sweet potato: *butternut squash*
> Quinoa: *brown rice or spelt*
> Hemp seeds: *sesame or chia seeds*
> Cashew nuts: *almonds or walnuts*

JACKFRUIT CAESAR SALAD

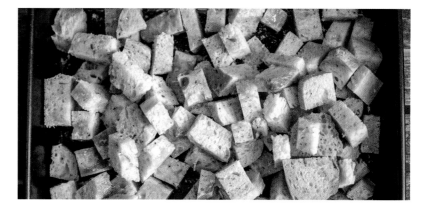

Serves: 4
Equipment: strainer, chopping board, kitchen paper, medium frying pan, medium baking tray, jug blender or a bowl and stick blender, very large serving bowl
Prep time: 20 minutes
Cooking time: 20 minutes

For the jackfruit:
560g/1¼lb young green canned jackfruit in brine (drained weight)
30ml/2 tbsp olive oil

For the croûtons:
45ml/3 tbsp olive oil
2 garlic cloves, finely chopped or crushed
4 thick slices of stale white bread, cut into 2.5cm/1in cubes

For the dressing:
300g/11oz silken tofu, drained
45ml/3 tbsp nutritional yeast
1 garlic clove, finely chopped
15ml/1 tbsp extra virgin olive oil
30ml/2 tbsp vegan mayonnaise
zest of ½ lemon and 22.5ml/1½ tbsp juice
5ml/1 tsp Dijon mustard
15ml/1 tbsp cider or white wine vinegar
5ml/1 tsp fine salt
1.25ml/¼ tsp ground black pepper
2.5ml/½ tsp sugar

For the salad:
2 heads romaine/cos lettuce, torn
4 spring onions (scallions), chopped
275g/10oz cherry tomatoes, halved

SUBSTITUTE INGREDIENTS
Jackfruit: *Quorn or Gardein chicken-style pieces*

Jackfruit does an incredible job of replicating the appearance and texture of chicken in this dish. It is slightly stringy, quite chewy, and doesn't have a strong flavour of its own, so takes on the Caesar dressing well. Just make sure to buy a tin of 'young green' jackfruit in brine, rather than ripe jackfruit in sweet syrup – somehow I don't think that would be as nice!

1 Preheat the oven to 200°C/400°F/Gas 6. Rinse the jackfruit in a strainer, then put it on a chopping board and pat dry with kitchen paper. Roughly chop the jackfruit and set aside. If you see a small, spherical piece of jackfruit, it's just a seed – these can be eaten.

2 Heat the olive oil in a medium frying pan over a medium heat. Sauté the jackfruit for 20 minutes, stirring occasionally. Set aside to cool.

3 While the jackfruit it cooking, heat the olive oil for the croûtons in a small frying pan over a medium-high heat. Fry the garlic for about 90 seconds, stopping if it's browning too quickly. Remove from the heat.

4 Spread the bread out on a medium baking tray. Pour the garlicky olive oil over the bread and mix well with your hands so all the bread is coated.

5 Bake the croûtons for 10–15 minutes, shaking halfway through, keeping an eye on them so they don't burn. Set aside.

6 Put all the dressing ingredients in a jug blender and blitz well until smooth. You could also do this with a bowl and a stick blender.

7 To assemble the salad, put the lettuce, spring onions and tomatoes in a very large serving bowl. Put the jackfruit on top, then pour over three-quarters of the dressing. Put the rest of the dressing in a small ramekin in case anyone wants extra. Mix the salad, add half the croûtons and gently mix them in. Finally, top with the rest of the croûtons and serve.

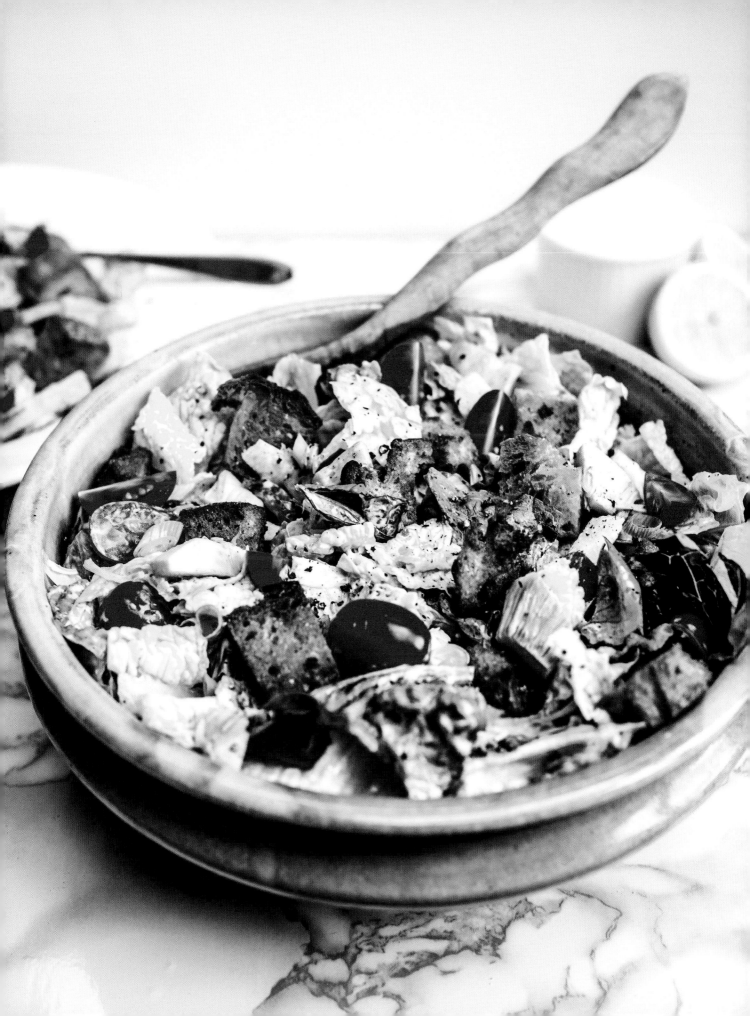

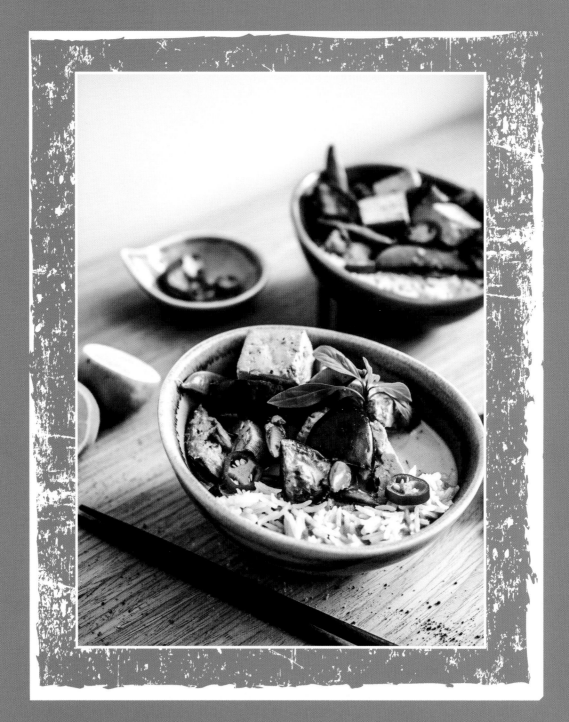

MAIN COURSES

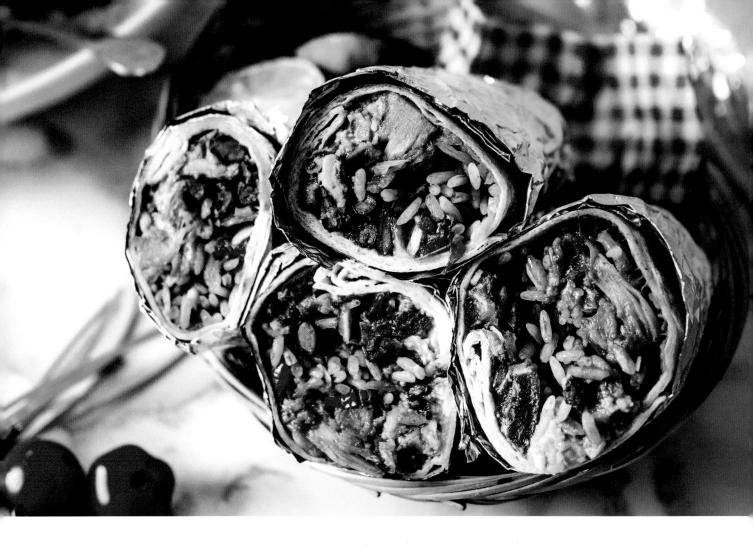

JUMBO JACKFRUIT BURRITOS

Salsa, guacamole, smoky home-made refried beans, vibrant Mexican rice and spicy, sweet-and-sour BBQ jackfruit come together in this epic burrito recipe. This is great to make for friends so that everyone assembles their own, Or, wrap a couple up, take them to work and count the minutes till lunch.

Serves: 4–6
Equipment: colander, bowl, chopping board, kitchen paper, large pan, non-stick medium pan with a lid, small bowl, potato masher or fork
Prep time: 30–40 minutes
Cooking time: about 40 minutes

For the pico de gallo:
500g/1¼lb ripe tomatoes, diced
2.5ml/½ tsp fine salt
½ medium red onion, diced
60ml/4 tbsp finely chopped fresh coriander (cilantro)
1 fresh green chilli, seeded and finely chopped (optional)
15ml/1 tbsp lime juice

1 For the pico de gallo, put the tomatoes in a colander set over a bowl and sprinkle all over with the salt. The excess moisture will start to drain out. Leave to drain for a minimum of 20 minutes.

2 Gently press down on the tomatoes with your hands to squeeze out the last of the juice. Discard the juice, then gently combine the tomato flesh with the onion, coriander, chilli and lime juice in the bowl. Set aside.

3 For the BBQ jackfruit, which you can make while the tomatoes are draining, rinse the jackfruit and drain it well, then put it on a chopping board and pat it dry with kitchen paper. Roughly chop the jackfruit and set it aside. If you see a small, spherical piece of jackfruit, it's just a seed – these can be eaten.

For the BBQ jackfruit:

560g/1¼lb young green canned jackfruit
in brine (drained weight)

45ml/3 tbsp neutral vegetable oil

1 medium onion, sliced

3 red (bell) peppers, sliced

15ml/1 tbsp smoked paprika

5ml/1 tsp ground cumin

a pinch of cayenne pepper

5ml/1 tsp dried oregano

1.25ml/¼ tsp ground black pepper

2.5ml/½ tsp yellow mustard seeds

175g/6oz/¾ cup tomato ketchup

7.5ml/½ tbsp soy sauce

7.5ml/½ tbsp cider vinegar

15ml/1 tbsp black treacle (molasses)

15ml/1 tbsp soft dark brown sugar

For the Mexican rice:

15ml/1 tbsp neutral vegetable oil

200g/7oz/1 cup long grain white
rice, rinsed

3 medium garlic cloves, sliced

7.5ml/1½ tsp tomato paste

2.5ml/½ tsp ground cumin

For the black beans:

22.5ml/1½ tbsp olive oil

2 medium garlic cloves, sliced

2.5ml/½ tsp cumin seeds

400g/14oz can black or pinto beans,
drained and rinsed

2.5ml/½ tsp smoked paprika

0.6ml/⅛ tsp fine salt

For the guacamole:

4 ripe avocados, scooped out and
roughly chopped

½ small onion, diced

1.25ml/¼ tsp fine salt

15ml/1 tbsp lime juice

8 large white flour tortillas

SUBSTITUTE INGREDIENTS

*If you don't have any black treacle use
molasses instead, or double the quantity
of soft dark brown sugar*

---

4 Heat the oil in a large pan over a medium-high heat. Add the sliced onion and peppers and fry for 10 minutes, stirring frequently. Add the smoked paprika, cumin, cayenne pepper, dried oregano, black pepper and mustard seeds, stir well and fry for 5 more minutes.

5 Add the jackfruit and mix until it's coated. Now add the tomato ketchup, soy sauce, vinegar, treacle and sugar and stir well. Bring to a boil, then reduce the heat to a low simmer and cook for 10 minutes. Set aside.

6 For the Mexican rice, which you can make while the BBQ jackfruit is simmering, heat the oil in a non-stick medium pan over a medium heat. Add the rice grains and fry for about 7 minutes, stirring occasionally, until golden brown. Add the garlic, tomato paste and cumin, stir well and fry for a few more minutes.

7 Add 420ml/15fl oz/1¾ cups water and bring to a boil. Turn the heat down to a low simmer, cover and cook until the water has been absorbed by the rice (about 15 minutes). Taste to check the rice is done. If not, add a little water and continue to cook until it is.

8 For the black beans, which you can make while the rice is simmering, heat the oil in a frying pan over high heat. Add the garlic and cumin seeds and fry for 2 minutes, then add the beans and smoked paprika and fry for 1–2 minutes more. Mix in the salt and set aside.

9 For the guacamole, put the avocado in a small bowl and use a potato masher or fork to mash. Mix in the onion and salt, then drizzle the lime juice over the surface of the guacamole to prevent it from browning while you assemble the burritos. Mix in the lime juice at the last minute.

10 To assemble, warm the tortillas slightly in the microwave or in a low oven. Spoon lines of jackfruit, rice, beans, pico de gallo and guacamole on a tortilla. Leave about a 2.5cm/1in space at the top and bottom.

11 Rotate the tortilla so the lines of filling are horizontal. Folding in each 2.5cm/1in end, lift the near edge of the wrap over the filling, then pull towards you slightly to tighten. Tightly roll the wrapped filling forwards and away from you to close. Repeat with the remaining tortillas.

12 If preparing for later, wrap the burrito in foil or clear film and store in the fridge. Otherwise, slice in half at a slight angle just before eating.

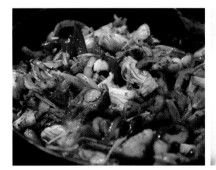 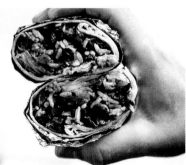

QUICK FALAFEL

Falafels are one of my favourite foods. I'll happily eat any type, from freshly fried ones at a trendy food truck to out-of-date, stale supermarket offerings. When making them myself, I've found the sacrifice in flavour that results from using canned chickpeas instead of dried is marginal – and using the former gives you the option to whip these up without prior planning. Which, let's face it, is how many of us cook.

Makes: 15 falafels
Equipment: food processor or jug blender or large bowl and stick blender, baking tray, large plate, kitchen paper, large, deep pan or deep-fat fryer, probe thermometer (optional) and slotted spoon OR large, non-stick frying pan OR baking tray
Prep time: 20 minutes, plus 30 minutes chilling
Cooking time: 15–25 minutes

2 handfuls (about 25g/1oz) fresh coriander (cilantro), stems and leaves, roughly chopped

2 handfuls (about 25g/1oz) fresh parsley, stems and leaves, roughly chopped

2 x 400g/14oz cans chickpeas, drained and patted dry

45ml/3 tbsp gram (chickpea) or plain (all-purpose) flour, plus extra for dusting

60ml/4 tbsp dried breadcrumbs

3 spring onions (scallions), whites and greens, chopped

2 medium garlic cloves, crushed

60ml/4 tbsp extra virgin olive oil

5ml/1 tsp ground cumin

5ml/1 tsp ground coriander

5ml/1 tsp fine salt

1.25ml/¼ tsp ground black pepper

475ml/16fl oz/2 cups sunflower oil (if deep-frying) or about 60ml/4 tbsp olive oil (if shallow-frying) or 45ml/3 tbsp olive oil (if baking)

To serve (optional):
hummus and/or Cashew Tzatziki (see page 58)
pitta bread or Middle Eastern Flatbreads (see page 151)
shredded lettuce and sliced tomatoes
sliced pickled beetroot (beets), pickled cabbage or gherkins
lemon wedges

1 Put all the ingredients apart from the cooking oil in a food processor or jug blender, or in a large bowl and use a stick blender, and blitz to a coarse paste. You may need to scrape down the sides.

2 Flour your hands and shape the mixture into about 15 balls. Transfer to a lightly floured baking tray and then place in the fridge for 30 minutes to firm up. Line a large plate with kitchen paper.

3 If shallow-frying, go to step 7. If baking, preheat the oven to 200°C/400°F/Gas 6, then go to step 8.

4 To deep-fry: heat the vegetable oil to 180°C/350°F over a medium heat in a large, deep pan or deep-fat fryer. To check the temperature without a probe thermometer, drop a cube of bread in the oil – it should be completely brown in 40–60 seconds.

5 Carefully lower the falafels into the oil using a slotted spoon. Don't overcrowd the pan; fry a maximum of half the falafels at once. Fry for 6–7 minutes, until a golden-brown crust has formed.

6 Remove the falafels with the slotted spoon to the paper-lined plate so the excess oil is absorbed. Now deep-fry the remaining falafels in the same way.

7 To shallow-fry: preheat the oven to 110°C/225°F/Gas ¼, heat the olive oil over a medium heat in a large, non-stick frying pan. Fry half of the falafels for 10–12 minutes, turning, until golden brown all over. Transfer to the kitchen paper-lined plate and keep warm in the oven. Now fry the remaining falafels (you may need to add a little more oil) in the same way.

8 To bake the falafels: put them on a baking tray and drizzle over the olive oil. Toss gently to coat, then bake in the preheated oven for 25 minutes.

9 Serve the falafels immediately, as a snack with some hummus and/or cashew tzatziki, or as a more substantial meal stuffed into pittas or flatbreads with lettuce, tomatoes, hummus, pickles and lemon wedges.

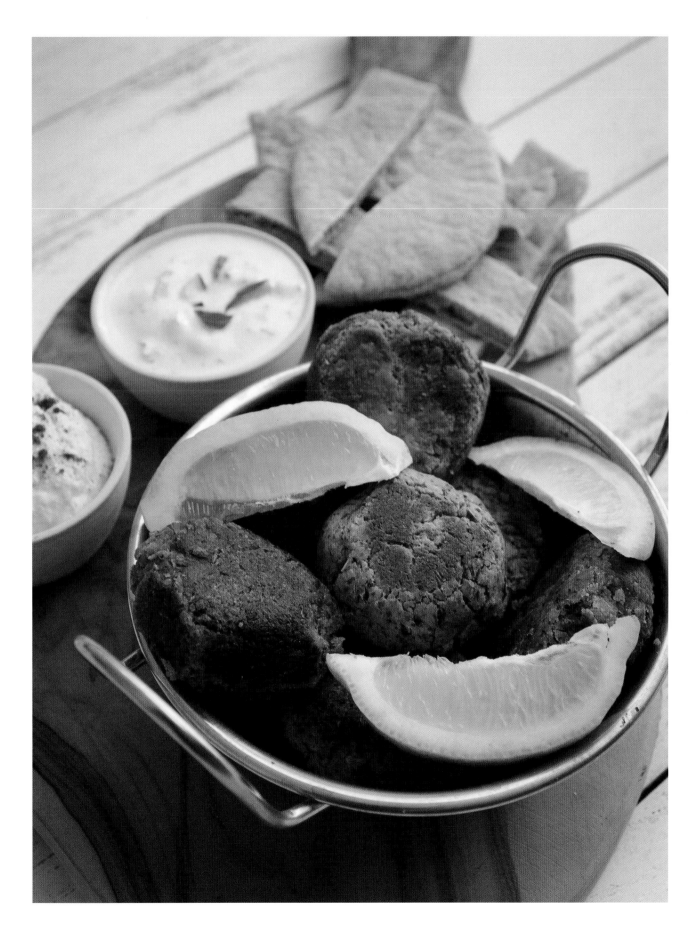

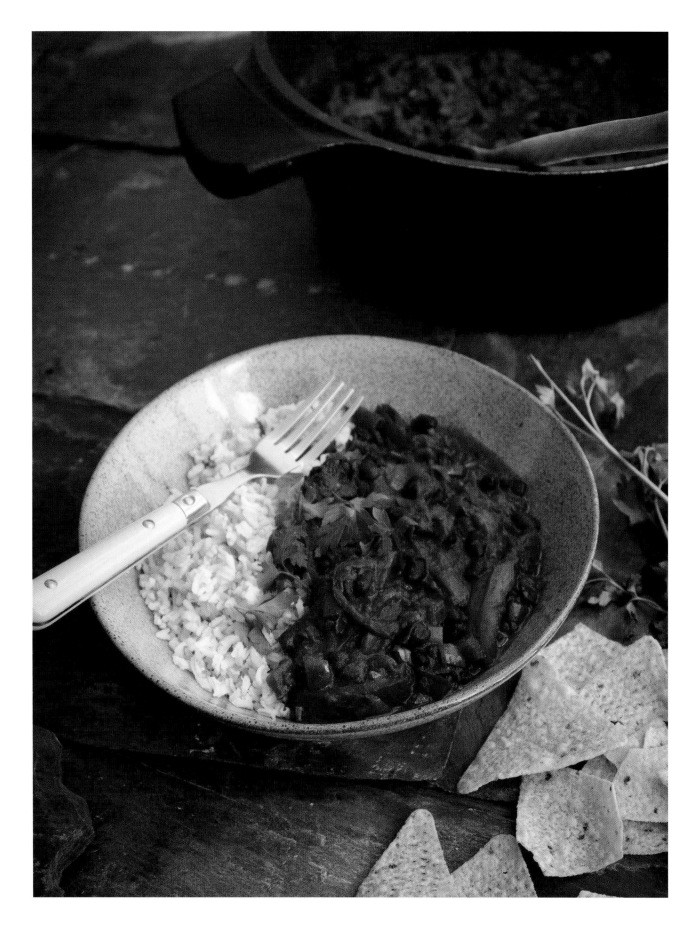

BLACK BEAN CHILLI SIN CARNE

Serves: 4
Equipment: large pan or casserole
Prep time: 15 minutes
Cooking time: 30–35 minutes

45ml/3 tbsp neutral vegetable oil

2 large red onions, chopped

1 large carrot, diced

2 Medjool dates, stoned (pitted) and finely chopped

30ml/2 tbsp ground cumin

30ml/2 tbsp smoked paprika

1.25ml/¼ tsp cayenne pepper

1 fresh jalapeño chilli, seeded and finely chopped

5 garlic cloves, finely chopped

4 Romano peppers, or 3 red (bell) peppers chopped into small strips

1 green (bell) pepper, chopped into small strips

2 x 400g/14oz cans chopped tomatoes

2 x 400g/14oz cans black beans, drained and rinsed

60ml/4 tbsp red wine

15g/½oz vegan dark (bittersweet) chocolate (optional)

60ml/4 tbsp red wine vinegar

10ml/2 tsp fine salt

2.5ml/½ tsp ground black pepper

fresh coriander (cilantro), to garnish

To serve:
Perfect Basmati Rice (see page 61)
tortilla chips (optional)

SUBSTITUTE INGREDIENTS
Medjool dates: *4 small dates or 5ml/1 tsp soft light brown sugar*
Black beans: *kidney beans*

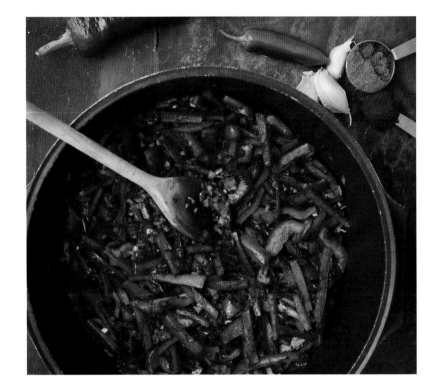

This smoky, spicy dish is what is what batch cooking is all about. It's filling, healthy and hearty, freezes well, and is easy to make. The chocolate is a traditional addition in Mexico and adds a dark, intense, full-bodied flavour to the dish, but is optional. You can add a few drops of liquid smoke to this recipe if you wish for an extra hickory hit.

1 Heat the oil in a large pan or casserole over a medium heat. Add the onions and carrot and sauté for 10 minutes, until starting to soften.

2 Add the dates, cumin, paprika and cayenne pepper and cook for 5 minutes.

3 Stir in the chilli, garlic and Romano and green peppers and cook for another 10 minutes, stirring occasionally.

4 Stir in the chopped tomatoes, black beans, red wine and chocolate, if using, and cook for 5–10 more minutes.

5 Stir in the vinegar, salt and ground black pepper.

6 Garnish with fresh coriander and serve with cooked rice and tortilla chips, if using, or store it in an airtight container – the flavour will only improve with a night in the fridge.

SUMMERY VEGETABLE RIGATONI

Here's two recipes for the price of one: the tomato sauce is fruity, peppery and made substantial with broken-down red lentils, and so versatile that it can be used for lots of other recipes besides this one, such as white bean stew, Epic Vegan Lasagne (see page 108) or even as a pizza sauce. You're welcome.

Serves: 4
Equipment: large pan or casserole, large frying pan, large pan, colander
Prep time: 20 minutes
Cooking time: 40 minutes

For the sauce:
60ml/4 tbsp olive oil
1 medium red onion, finely chopped
1 medium white onion, finely chopped
4 large garlic cloves, finely chopped
15ml/1 tbsp dried oregano
10ml/2 tsp dried thyme
5ml/1 tsp sugar
100g/3¾oz/½ cup dried red lentils, rinsed
2 x 400g/14oz chopped tomatoes
7.5ml/1½ tsp fine salt
2.5ml/½ tsp freshly ground black pepper
30ml/2 tbsp olive oil
3 medium courgettes (zucchini), chopped
250g/9oz chestnut mushrooms, halved
350g/12oz dried rigatoni
12 large basil leaves, torn, to garnish

1 For the sauce, heat the oil in a large pan or casserole over a medium heat. Add the onions and sauté for 5 minutes. Add the garlic and cook for 5 minutes, then stir in the oregano, thyme and sugar and cook for 2 minutes.

2 Stir in the lentils, followed by the chopped tomatoes. Fill one of the empty cans with water and add that, too. Leave to simmer for 25 minutes, then stir in the salt and ground black pepper.

3 Meanwhile, heat the oil in a large frying pan over a medium-high heat. Add the courgettes and mushrooms and fry for 10–12 minutes. The pan will be a little crowded but the mushrooms will cook down. The courgettes shouldn't be crunchy, but not too mushy either.

4 While the sauce and vegetables are cooking, bring a large pan of salted water to the boil. Add the pasta, bring back to a boil, then reduce the heat to a simmer and cook for 1 minute less than the packet says for al dente pasta. Drain in a colander, reserving 120ml/4fl oz/½ cup pasta water for later use.

5 When everything has finished cooking, stir the vegetables and pasta into the tomato sauce. If the sauce is looking a little dry, add some of the reserved pasta water to loosen.

6 Sprinkle over the basil leaves then serve with an extra grind of black pepper, if you like.

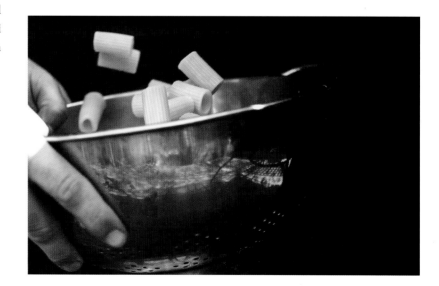

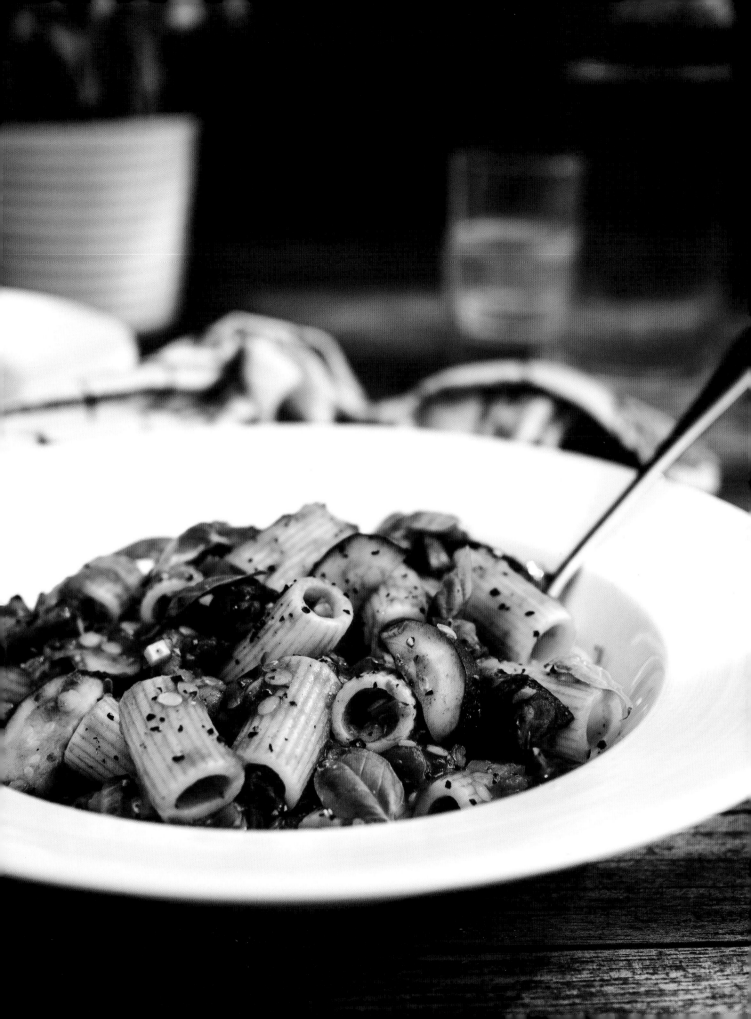

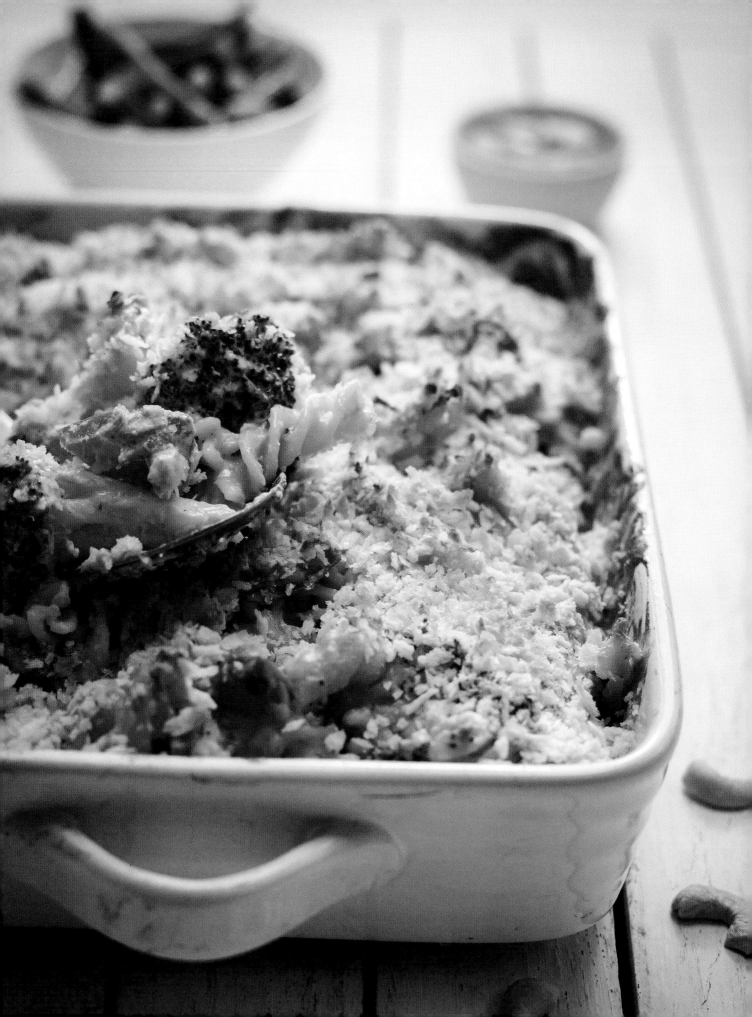

PASTA BAKE WITH CREAMY CASHEW SAUCE

The name 'pasta bake' reminds me of my secondary school's offering; a rubbery cuboid, more suitable as a basketball than food to be eaten for lunch. Anyway, do rest assured this recipe is nothing like that; cashews are used to create a luxuriously creamy, smooth sauce with a little kick from Dijon mustard and cheesiness from nutritional yeast flakes, which coats the pasta and veg to produce a nourishing all-in-one meal.

Serves: 3–4
Equipment: small bowl, strainer, jug blender or food processor, large pan, deep ovenproof dish (about 30 x 20 x 7.5cm/12 x 8 x 3in)
Prep time: 15 minutes, plus 15 minutes soaking
Cooking time: 30–40 minutes

175g/6oz/1 cup unsalted, unroasted cashews
250ml/8fl oz/1 cup unsweetened soya milk
15ml/1 tbsp lemon juice
10ml/2 tsp Dijon mustard
60ml/4 tbsp nutritional yeast
1.25ml/¼ tsp ground nutmeg
3.75ml/¾ tsp fine salt
1.25ml/¼ tsp ground black pepper
200g/7oz/scant 2 cups dried fusilli
200g/7oz broccoli florets
4 ripe medium tomatoes, roughly chopped
45g/1½oz/½ cup fresh breadcrumbs

1 Preheat the oven to 180°C/350°F/Gas 4.

2 Put the cashews in a small bowl, pour over boiling water to cover and leave to soak for 15 minutes, until softened and swollen.

3 Drain the cashews and place them in a blender (or, less preferably, a food processor). Add 60ml/4 tbsp of the soya milk and blend for about 2 minutes or until very smooth. Keep blending if it's still at all granular.

4 Add the lemon juice, mustard, nutritional yeast, nutmeg, salt, ground black pepper and the remaining soya milk and blend again until smooth. You should have a thick, creamy sauce.

5 Bring 2 litres/3½ pints/8 cups salted water to a boil in a large pan. Add the pasta and bring back to a boil. Reduce the heat and simmer until al dente (use packet instructions for timing). Add the broccoli florets to the simmering pasta for the last 4 minutes of cooking.

6 Drain the pasta and broccoli, then transfer to the deep ovenproof dish. Add the chopped tomatoes and gently stir to distribute evenly. Pour over the cashew sauce and stir gently to combine.

7 Sprinkle the breadcrumbs on top and bake for 20–30 minutes, until bubbling and golden.

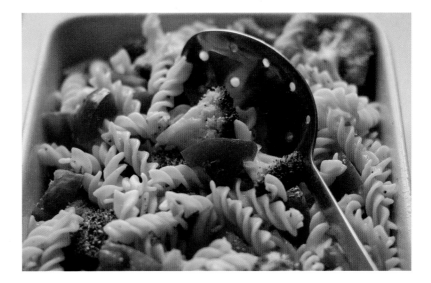

SUBSTITUTE INGREDIENTS
Fusilli: *elbow macaroni or penne*
Broccoli: *cauliflower*
Soya milk: *any unsweetened plant milk*
Dijon mustard: *wholegrain mustard*

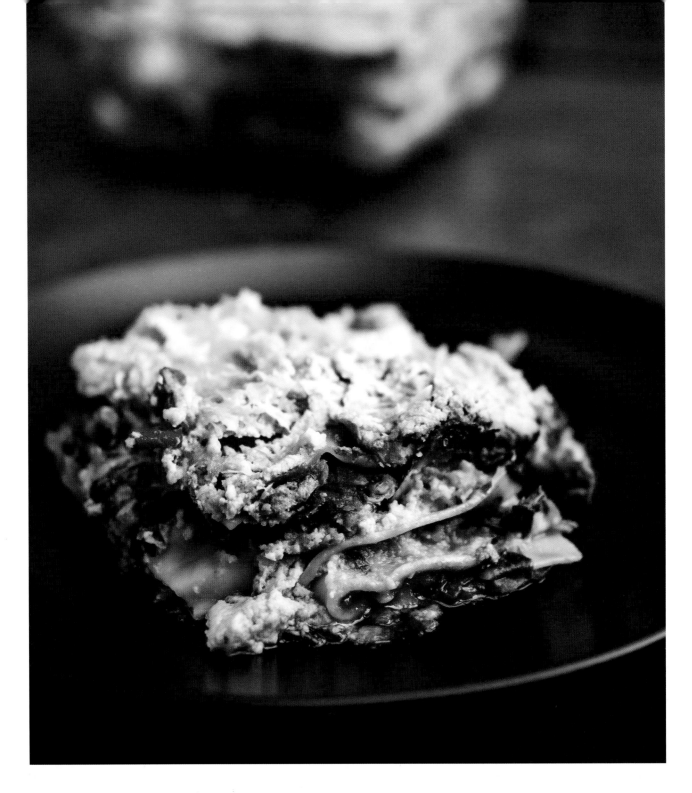

EPIC VEGAN LASAGNE

Everyone loves this dish. My aunt *doubled* the already large proportions to feed 12 hungry sailors. Celeriac, steamed and blitzed with a generous amount of olive oil, makes an excellent and surprisingly creamy 'béchamel'. The tomato and red lentil sauce is certainly no mere filler, either – it's fruity, warming and flavoured with plenty of oregano and thyme that screams *Italian!*

Serves: 4–6
Equipment: large frying pan, steamer basket and pan, colander, food processor or jug blender or bowl and stick blender, 2 baking trays, 3½ litre/6 pint/15-cup ovenproof baking dish (rim roughly 28 x 21cm/11 x 8½in), foil, freezer bag and rolling pin (optional), small bowl
Prep time: 40 minutes, plus 5–10 minutes standing
Cooking time: 1 hour 30 minutes

For the tomato-lentil sauce:

45ml/3 tbsp olive oil
1 medium red onion, finely chopped
1 medium white onion, finely chopped
4 large garlic cloves, finely chopped
1 medium fresh red chilli, seeded and thinly sliced
1 red (bell) pepper, chopped
15ml/1 tbsp dried oregano
10ml/2 tsp dried thyme
5ml/1 tsp fine salt
5ml/1 tsp sugar
225g/8oz/1 cup dried red lentils, rinsed
2 x 400ml/14oz cans chopped tomatoes
a good grind of ground black pepper

For the celeriac 'béchamel':

1 medium (roughly 600g/1lb 6oz) celeriac (celery root), peeled and chopped
120ml/4fl oz/½ cup extra virgin olive oil
2.5ml/½ tsp fine salt

To assemble:

200g/7oz lasagne sheets
15ml/1 tbsp neutral vegetable oil, for greasing
175g/6oz baby or leaf spinach, finely chopped
3 large handfuls (about 115g/4oz) of tortilla chips
45g/1½oz/½ cup dried breadcrumbs

1 First, make the tomato-lentil sauce. Heat the oil in a large frying pan over a medium heat. Add the onions and sauté for 5 minutes, then add the garlic, chilli and the pepper and cook for 10 more minutes.

2 Stir in the oregano, thyme, salt, sugar and lentils, followed by the chopped tomatoes. Fill one of the empty cans with water and add that, too. Leave to simmer for 25 minutes, then add the black pepper and set aside.

3 While the sauce is cooking, steam the celeriac over a pan of simmering water for 15 minutes, until it's soft but not mushy. Cool the celeriac down by rinsing it thoroughly with cold water. Shake it to ensure it is drained, then place it in a food processor or jug blender, and blitz to a purée.

4 With the food processor motor still running, very slowly drizzle in the olive oil, so it is well incorporated into the celeriac purée. If you are using a jug or stick blender instead of a food processor, add the oil 15ml/1 tbsp at a time in between pulses. Add the salt and pulse one more time. Set aside.

5 Preheat the oven to 180°C/350°F/Gas 4. Boil 500ml/17fl oz/generous 2 cups water in the kettle. Lay the lasagne sheets out in a single layer on 2 baking trays. Pour the boiling water over the lasagne sheets and soak for 2–3 minutes, then drain the water.

6 To assemble, grease an ovenproof baking dish with oil, then pour one-third of the tomato-lentil sauce into the base of the dish. Cover with a layer of lasagne sheets, then spread over half the celeriac 'béchamel'. Sprinkle half of the spinach on top, then another third of tomato-lentil sauce and then another layer of lasagne sheets. Repeat the layers, finishing with béchamel, then cover with foil and bake for 40 minutes.

7 Meanwhile, blitz the tortilla chips in a food processor to a breadcrumb consistency. Alternatively, put them in a freezer bag and crush them with a rolling pin. Combine with the breadcrumbs in a small bowl.

8 After the lasagne has been in the oven for 40 minutes, take it out and uncover it. Evenly sprinkle the breadcrumbs and crushed tortilla chips over the surface. Return to the oven for 10 minutes, until golden. Remove from the oven and leave to stand for 5–10 minutes before serving.

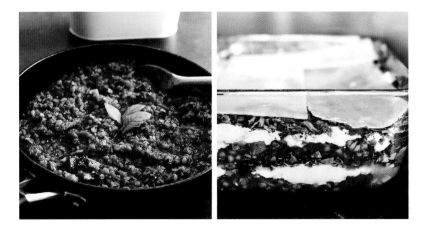

MUSHROOM RISOTTO

I'll come clean: I've always found it hard to get excited about risotto. 'Too much fuss over clumpy rice', said me, before writing this book. But after numerous recipe tests, the challenge has brought with it a certain appreciation. What was previously a bowl of stodgy rice has become a labour of love: elegant grains plump with rich porcini mushroom stock, white wine and olive oil.

Serves: 4
Equipment: small bowl, wide, tall-sided frying pan or casserole, strainer, small pan
Prep time: 15 minutes
Cooking time: 30–40 minutes

15 medium (about 10g/¼oz) dried porcini mushroom pieces, roughly chopped
45ml/3 tbsp olive oil
2 medium shallots, very finely chopped
3 large garlic cloves, finely chopped or crushed
300g/11oz/1½ cups Arborio or carnaroli rice
175ml/6fl oz/¾ cup white wine
350g/12oz chestnut mushrooms, chopped
5ml/1 tsp fine salt
1.25ml/¼ tsp ground black pepper
30ml/2 tbsp finely chopped fresh parsley
grated vegan Parmesan cheese, to serve (optional)

1 Put the porcini mushrooms into a small bowl, pour over 250ml/8fl oz/1 cup boiling water, and set aside.

2 Heat the oil in a wide, tall-sided frying pan or casserole over a medium heat. Add the shallots and garlic to the pan and sauté for 10 minutes. Stir the rice in well and cook gently for 5 minutes.

3 Strain the soaked porcini into a small pan, reserving the soaking liquid, and add the strained porcini to the rice mixture.

4 Pour the wine into the porcini soaking liquid, place over a medium heat and bring to a boil, then turn down to a very low simmer.

5 Ladle 300ml/½ pint/1¼ cups of the hot wine and stock into the rice. Cook, stirring constantly, until the rice has absorbed most of the liquid. Ladle another 300ml/½ pint/1¼ cups of the hot wine and stock into the rice and keep stirring until it has been absorbed.

6 Add the chestnut mushrooms to the rice, then ladle in 300ml/½ pint/1¼ cups more wine/stock, stirring until absorbed, until there's no stock left, and the rice is plump and cooked through. This will take about 15 minutes, but do test it as the rice can vary. Meanwhile, warm four wide serving bowls.

7 Stir the salt and ground black pepper into the risotto along with most of the parsley. Leave to rest for a couple of minutes. Ladle the risotto into the warm bowls, sprinkle over the reserved parsley and grate over some vegan Parmesan cheese, if using.

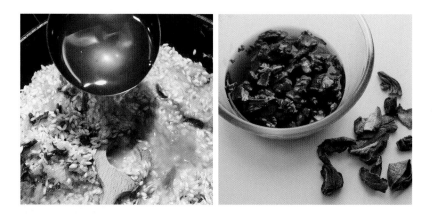

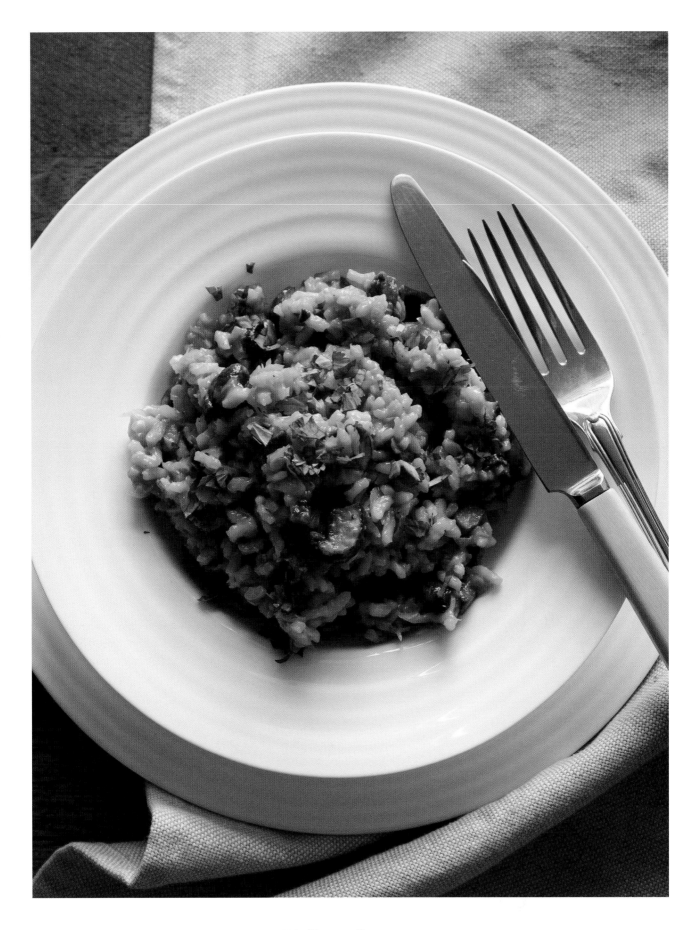

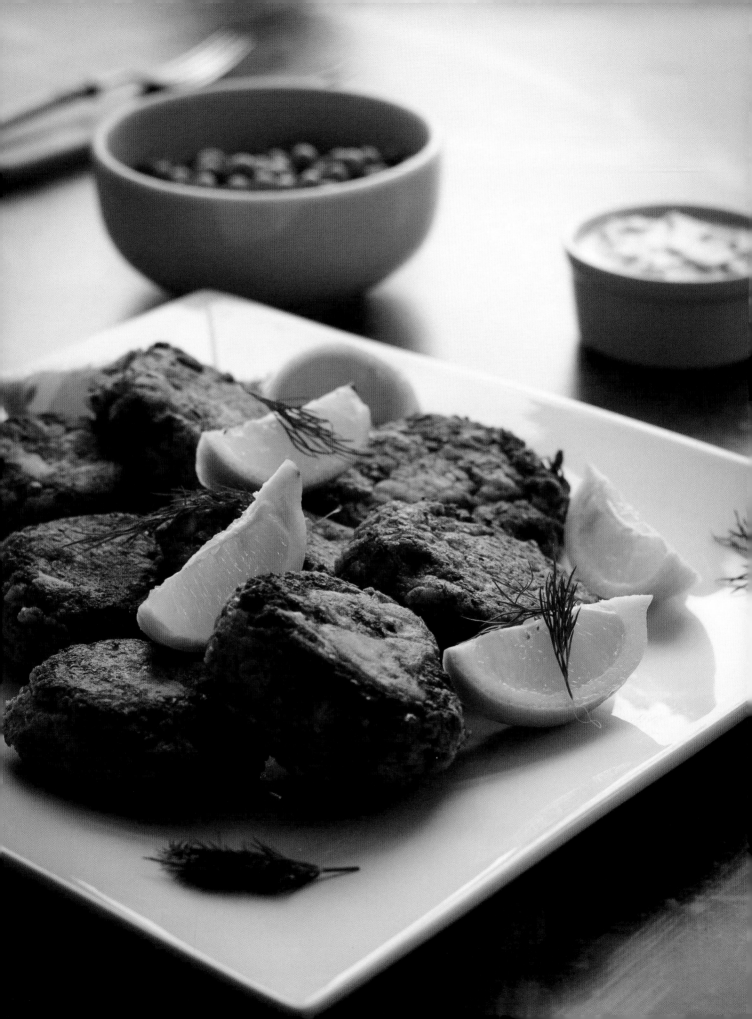

'FISH' CAKES

When I wrote this recipe, I hoped these 'fish' cakes would have a hint of fish. I asked my dad to rate their fishiness from 1–10, hoping for a three. On tasting them myself, I paused the TV, shocked. 'Well?! Score?' He gave them an eight, mystified. I hadn't anticipated how much of the flavour in fish comes from their omega-3 oils, and since flaxseeds (also called linseeds) contain an abundance of these omega-3s, and toasting them coaxes out this flavour, the end result is surprisingly fishy.

Makes: 8 cakes
Equipment: medium pan with a lid, colander, small frying pan, small bowl, large bowl, 2 plates, clear film (plastic wrap) or a damp dish towel, 1 large or 2 small baking trays or a wide, non-stick frying pan
Prep time: 30 minutes, plus thickening time
Cooking time: about 30 minutes

400g/14oz floury potatoes, peeled and cubed
30ml/2 tbsp ground flaxseeds/linseeds
2 medium nori sheets
400g/14oz can chickpeas, drained and patted dry
30ml/2 tbsp plain (all-purpose) flour, plus extra for dusting
45ml/3 tbsp dried breadcrumbs
5ml/1 tsp dried thyme
15ml/1 tbsp onion granules, dried onions or onion powder
5ml/1 tsp fine salt
1.25ml/¼ tsp ground black pepper
1.25ml/¼ tsp ground white pepper
2 spring onions (scallions), white and greens, sliced
45ml/3 tbsp tomato ketchup
30ml/2 tbsp vegan mayonnaise
45ml/3 tbsp lemon juice
45ml/3 tbsp vegetable oil (if frying)

To serve (optional):
Tartare Sauce (see page 32)
tomato ketchup
peas, or steamed greens
lemon wedges

1 Put the potatoes in a medium pan, cover with water and put on the lid. Bring to a boil, then remove the lid, turn the heat down to a simmer and cook for 10 minutes or until soft. Drain well in a colander.

2 Meanwhile, put the ground flaxseeds/linseeds in a small frying pan over a medium-high heat. Toast for 7–8 minutes, tossing regularly, until their colour deepens and they give off a fish-like aroma.

3 Transfer the toasted seeds to a small bowl and stir in 90ml/6 tbsp water. Set aside for 15 minutes to thicken into a gel.

4 Roughly crumble the nori sheets into a large bowl, then add the chickpeas, flour, breadcrumbs, thyme, onion granules, salt, ground black and white pepper, spring onions, ketchup, mayonnaise and lemon juice. Stir to combine.

5 Add the cooked potatoes and flaxseed/linseed gel to the bowl and mash everything to a chunky, cohesive mixture using a potato masher. Tip the mixture on to a floured surface and divide into 8 portions.

7 Sprinkle two plates with flour, then flour your hands and shape the divided mixture into round, 2.5cm/1in-thick patties. Place 4 cakes on each plate and cover loosely with clear film or a damp dish towel. Chill in the fridge for 30 minutes. You could freeze all or half of the cakes at this point.

8 Preheat the oven to 110°C/220°F/Gas ¼ . Heat the oil in a wide, non-stick frying pan over a medium heat. Fry 4 cakes for 6 minutes on one side and 4 minutes on the other, until golden brown. Transfer back to the plate and keep warm in the oven while you fry the other cakes.

9 Serve with vegan tartare sauce, ketchup, peas or steamed greens and lemon wedges.

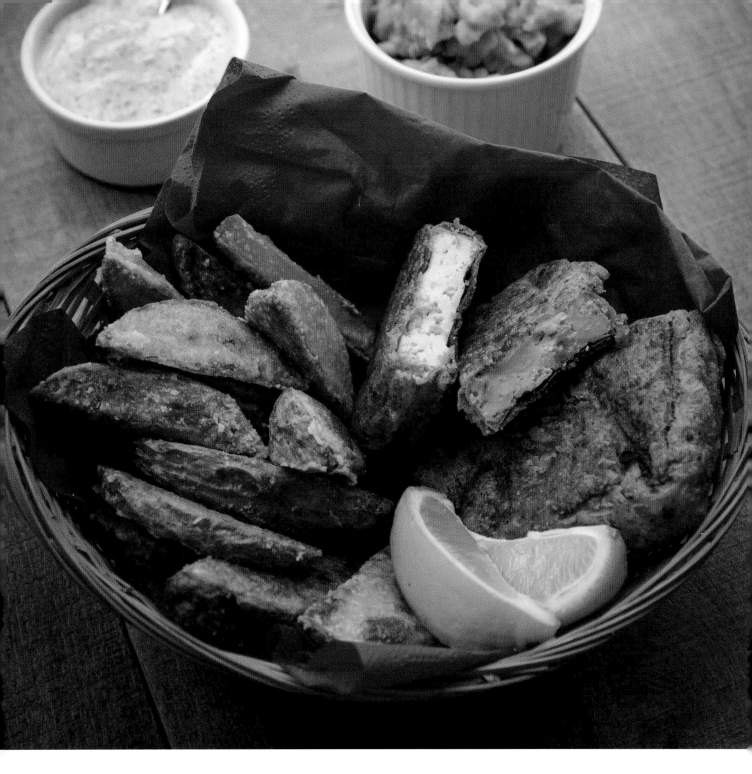

TOFU 'FISH' 'N' CHIPS

The idea may sound amusing, but there are even bespoke 'tofu 'n' chips' shops opening now. Beer gives the batter a deeper flavour and helps achieve a light, crisp exterior, though sparkling water works well, too, as in tempura batter. Similar to the 'fish' cakes on page 113, this recipe takes advantage of the omega-3 oils in flaxseeds/linseeds to provide a fishy flavour and aroma. Baking the chips rather than deep-frying them will ensure everything is hot at the same time.

Serves: 4
Equipment: kitchen paper or clean dish towels, heavy weight, large baking tray, small frying pan, large plate, kitchen paper, large, deep pan or deep-fat fryer, probe thermometer (optional), medium bowl, whisk, slotted spoon or tongs
Prep time: 30 minutes, plus 30 minutes pressing
Cooking time: about 30 minutes

For the tofu:

800g/1¾lb extra-firm tofu, drained
60ml/4 tbsp ground flaxseeds/linseeds
2 x 15 x 20cm/6 x 8in nori sheets
475ml/16fl oz/2 cups sunflower oil, for deep-frying
7.5ml/1½ tsp baking powder
5ml/1 tsp fine salt
175g/6oz/1½ cups plain (all-purpose) flour
750ml/1¼ pints/3 cups cold fizzy lager or sparkling water

For the chips:

600g/1lb 6oz floury potatoes, cut into 1cm/½in-thick wedges
2.5ml/½ tsp fine salt
40g/1½oz/⅓ cup cornflour (corn starch)
90ml/6 tbsp neutral vegetable oil

To serve (optional):

steamed, boiled or mushy peas
tomato ketchup
Tartare Sauce (see page 32)
lemon wedges

1 Preheat the oven to 200°C/400°F/Gas 6. Place several layers of kitchen paper towels, or a couple of clean dish towels, on a plate. Put the tofu on the towels and cover with more paper/dish towels. Place a heavy object, such as a book or a heavy pan, on top to press the water out of the tofu. Leave to drain for at least 30 minutes. If you're short of time, press down on the heavy object to get as much water out of the tofu as possible.

2 For the chips, put the potatoes on a large baking tray. Sprinkle over the salt and cornflour and gently toss so all the wedges are coated. Drizzle over the oil and briefly toss again. Bake for 25 minutes, until golden brown. If the chips are done before you've finished frying the tofu, turn the oven off, leaving the chips inside to keep warm.

3 While the chips are cooking, carefully split each pressed tofu block sideways through the middle, then cut each piece diagonally into two, so that you have eight triangular 'fillets'.

4 Toast the ground flaxseeds/linseeds in a small frying pan over a medium-high heat for 7–8 minutes, tossing regularly, until their colour deepens and they give off a fishy aroma. Set aside.

5 Cut each nori sheet into four pieces and apply one to the back of each tofu 'fillet' as the fish 'skin'. Line a large plate with kitchen paper.

6 Heat the vegetable oil to 180°C/350°F over a medium heat in a large, deep pan or deep-fat fryer. To check the temperature without a probe thermometer, drop a cube of bread in the oil – it should be completely brown in 40–60 seconds.

7 While the oil is heating up, make the batter. Stir the toasted flaxseeds/linseeds, baking powder and salt into the flour in a medium bowl. Gradually whisk in the lager or sparkling water to form a smooth batter.

8 Submerge a tofu fillet in the batter, then lower it into the hot oil using a slotted spoon or tongs. Be careful as the hot oil may splutter. Batter and fry several tofu fillets at the same time, if your pan/fryer is large enough. Fry for 5–7 minutes until a golden brown, crisp outer layer has formed.

9 Transfer the fried tofu to the kitchen paper to drain off the excess oil. If you need to fry in two batches, keep the cooked fillets warm on a baking tray. Serve with the chips, peas, ketchup, tartare sauce and lemon wedges.

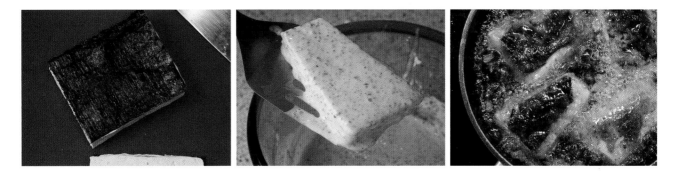

PROPER VEGGIE BURGERS

Makes: 8 burgers
Equipment: medium pan with a lid, kitchen paper, small pan with a lid, strainer, baking tray, medium frying pan, food processor or blender, large bowl, fork, 2 plates or trays, baking parchment, clear film (plastic wrap) or a damp dish towel, wide, non-stick frying pan, baking tray
Prep time: 30–40 minutes, plus 30 minutes chilling
Cooking time: about 45 minutes

300g/11oz potatoes, peeled and cubed
100g/3¾oz/½ cup pearl barley
400g/14oz can chickpeas or black beans, drained and patted dry
90ml/6 tbsp olive oil
250g/9oz button (white) or chestnut mushrooms, chopped
1 medium onion, finely chopped
1 red (bell) pepper, finely chopped
3 garlic cloves, finely chopped
30ml/2 tbsp plain (all-purpose) flour, plus extra for dusting
22.5ml/1½ tbsp lemon juice
45ml/3 tbsp sunflower seeds
15ml/1 tbsp soy sauce
5ml/1 tsp yeast extract
50g/2oz/1 cup fresh breadcrumbs
5ml/1 tsp fine salt
2.5ml/½ tsp ground black pepper
2.5ml/½ tsp ground cumin
2.5ml/½ tsp ground coriander
5ml/1 tsp smoked paprika
120ml/4fl oz/½ cup coconut oil
45ml/3 tbsp polenta
8 burger buns
tomato ketchup, mustard, red onion rings, tomato slices, lettuce leaves and sliced gherkins, to serve

Making good veggie burgers can be tricky without the saturated fat in beef or an egg to act as a binder. This recipe gets around those problems by using coconut oil for a juicy texture, a potato and chickpea flour purée as a binder, and mushrooms, soy sauce and yeast extract for an umami hit. Sunflower seeds, pearl barley and roasted chickpeas provide a nubbly texture, and a crust is achieved with polenta.

1 Preheat the oven to 180°C/350°F/Gas 4. Put the potatoes in a medium pan and cover with water. Bring to a boil, then simmer for 10 minutes or until soft. Strain, then transfer to sheets of kitchen paper to dry.

2 Meanwhile, put the barley in another small pan and add water to cover by about 2.5cm/1in. Cover with a lid, bring to a boil, then simmer for 25 minutes. Strain, then transfer to sheets of kitchen paper to dry.

3 While the barley is cooking, put half of the chickpeas or beans on a baking tray and roast in the oven for 20–25 minutes. At the same time, heat 45ml/3 tbsp of the olive oil in a medium frying pan over a medium heat. Add the mushrooms and sauté for 15 minutes or until the liquid has evaporated. Add the onion, red pepper and garlic and cook for 15 more minutes.

4 In a food processor or blender, blitz the remaining chickpeas with the flour, lemon juice and remaining 45ml/3 tbsp olive oil to a smooth paste. Add the potatoes and blitz again. Transfer this mixture to a large bowl.

5 Add the cooked barley, onions, peppers and mushrooms, chickpeas, sunflower seeds, soy sauce, yeast extract, breadcrumbs, salt, ground black pepper, cumin, coriander, paprika and 45ml/3 tbsp of the coconut oil to the chickpea-potato mixture. Mix thoroughly to combine.

6 Transfer the mixture back to the food processor or blender. Pulse about 10 times, for a chunky consistency. Preheat the oven to 140°C/275°F/Gas 1.

7 Line a baking tray with baking parchment and sprinkle on 30ml/2 tbsp of the polenta. Flour your hands and form the mixture into 8 patties, then place on the lined tray. Sprinkle the remaining polenta on top of each burger, cover loosely with a damp dish towel, and chill for 30 minutes.

8 Heat 45ml/3 tbsp of the coconut oil in a wide frying pan over a medium-high heat. Fry 4 burgers at a time for 6 minutes, then flip and fry for 4 more minutes. Transfer to a baking tray and keep warm in the oven while you fry the remaining burgers in the rest of the coconut oil.

9 Toast the buns, if you like, then serve the burgers with the various accompaniments, letting people mix and match their own combinations.

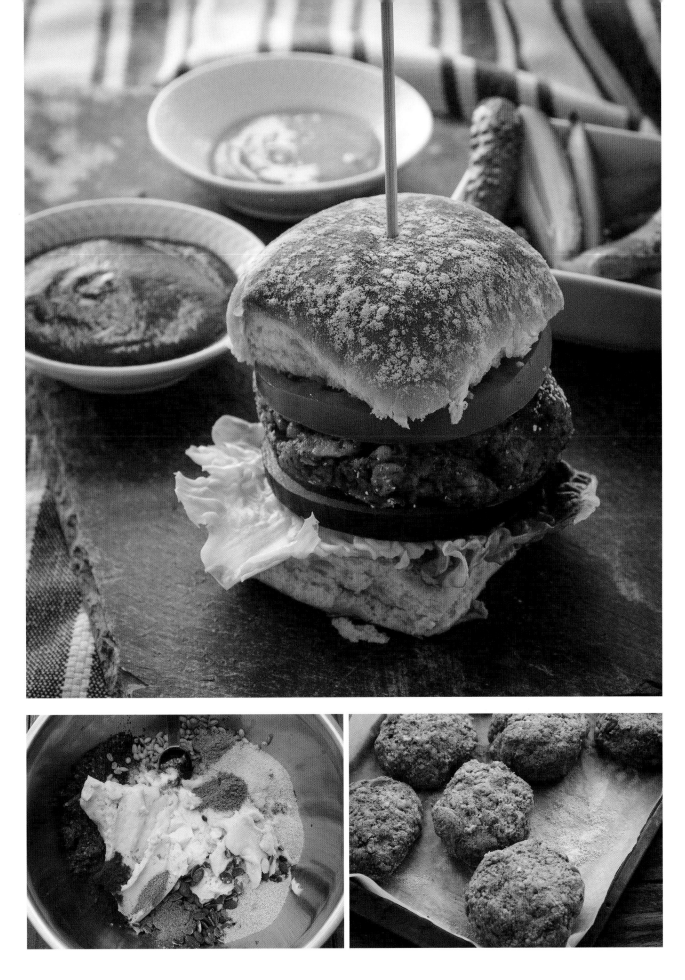

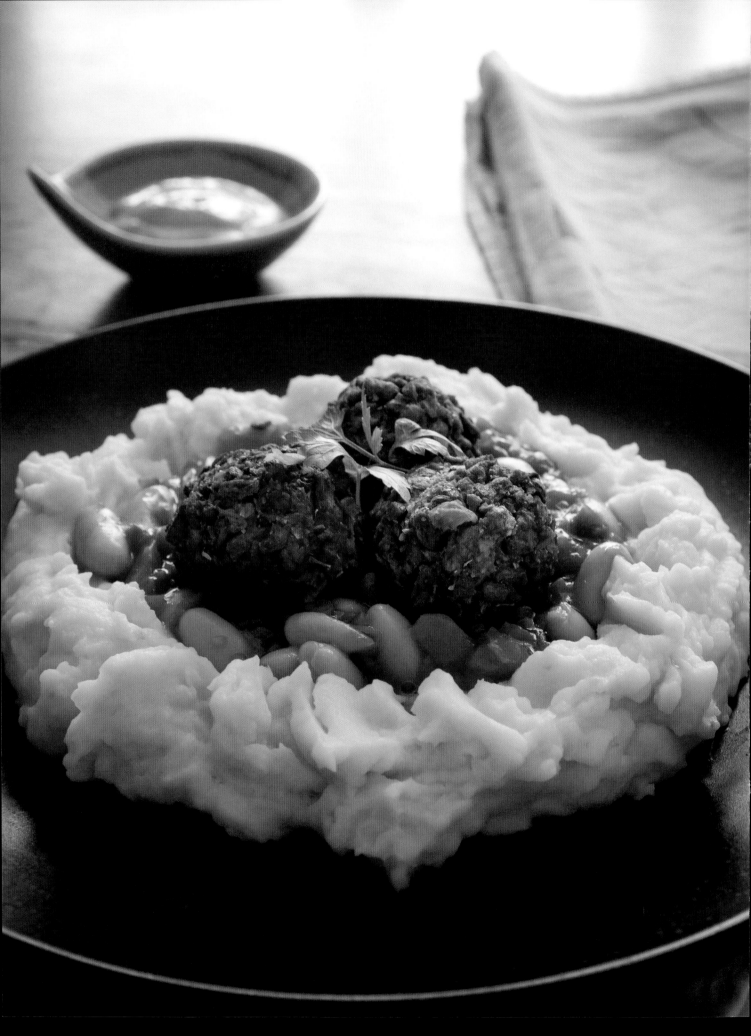

'MEATBALLS', MASH, & GRAVY

Serves: 4–6 (makes 20–24 'meatballs')
Equipment: small bowl, 2 large frying pans, large bowl, large baking tray, clear film (plastic wrap) or a damp dish towel, large pan, colander, potato masher
Prep time: 30 minutes, plus 15 minutes thickening and 25 minutes chilling
Cooking time: about 40 minutes

45ml/3 tbsp ground flaxseeds/linseeds
105ml/7 tbsp olive oil
1 large carrot, finely chopped
1 medium onion, finely chopped
2 garlic cloves, finely chopped
1 sage leaf, torn into a few pieces
500g/1¼lb frozen vegan meat-free mince
1.25ml/¼ tsp ground black pepper
1.25ml/¼ tsp ground white pepper
0.6ml/⅛ tsp ground nutmeg
5ml/1 tsp dried oregano
2.5ml/¼ tsp dried thyme
5ml/1 tsp fine salt
flour, for dusting
75ml/5 tbsp fresh breadcrumbs
mustard, to serve (optional)

For the bean gravy:
45ml/3 tbsp vegan onion gravy granules
400g/14oz can cannellini beans, drained

For the mash:
500g/1¼lb floury potatoes (e.g. King Edward), peeled and cut into even pieces
45ml/3 tbsp olive oil
60ml/4 tbsp unsweetened plant milk
salt and ground black pepper, to taste

There's something elegant about this crudely named dish. It took me several attempts to make a 'meatball' that wouldn't count as a disservice to their rich history in Italian cooking. I tried various binders, but ground flaxseeds produced the goods again. I'm particularly fond of the spice mix; white pepper, sage and nutmeg don't generally feature in my cooking but here they go together extremely well.

1 Mix the ground flaxseeds/linseeds with 110ml/3½fl oz/scant ½ cup water in a small bowl and set aside for 15 minutes to thicken into a gel.

2 Heat 60ml/4 tbsp of the oil in a large frying pan over a medium heat. Add the carrot, onion, garlic and sage and sauté for 10 minutes. Set aside half of the sautéed vegetables for the gravy.

3 Add the meat-free mince to the frying pan and sauté for 5 minutes, then transfer to a large bowl. Mix in the black and white pepper, ground nutmeg, oregano, thyme and salt, then add the breadcrumbs and flaxseed/linseed gel and mix thoroughly.

4 Sprinkle a large baking tray with flour and flour or dampen your hands. Shape 30ml/2 tbsp-sized pieces of the mixture into balls. Transfer the shaped 'meatballs' to the floured tray and cover loosely with clear film or a damp dish towel. Put the tray in the fridge and chill for at least 25 minutes.

5 Meanwhile, make the gravy. Put the gravy granules and 250ml/8fl oz/ 1 cup water in the frying pan in which you cooked the mince, along with the reserved sautéed vegetables. Bring to a boil, then turn down the heat and simmer for 5 minutes. Stir in the cannellini beans.

6 Preheat the oven to 110°C/225°F/Gas ¼. For the mash, boil the potatoes in a large pan for 15–20 minutes (depending on the size of the pieces), until soft.

7 Meanwhile, in a clean large frying pan, heat the remaining 45ml/3 tbsp olive oil over a medium heat. Fry as many 'meatballs' as will comfortably fit for 10–12 minutes, until golden brown all over. Transfer back to the baking tray and keep warm in the oven while you fry the remaining 'meatballs' in the same way.

8 Drain the cooked potatoes well in a colander, then mash with the olive oil and plant milk. Season to taste with salt and ground black pepper.

9 Serve the mash into wide bowls. Top with a few 'meatballs' and spoon over a generous amount of the bean-gravy, and serve with some mustard on the side, if you like.

CLASSIC 'CHICKEN' & MUSHROOM PIE

It was a pleasant surprise to find out that it is possible to buy ready-made vegan puff pastry in supermarkets – and so the door to savoury and sweet pies is wide open. Vegan 'chicken', cooked in a pie, is nearly indistinguishable from real chicken in my opinion. Fresh tarragon, which I don't often cook with, pairs perfectly with the savoury flavours of the filling.

Serves: 4
Equipment: baking sheet, 23 x 20cm/9 x 8in pie dish, large, wide pan or casserole, rolling pin, whisk, small bowl, pastry brush
Prep time: 30 minutes, plus cooling
Cooking time: 1 hour 15 minutes

45ml/3 tbsp neutral vegetable oil, plus extra for greasing
250g/9oz white or chestnut mushrooms, chopped
1 large carrot, finely chopped
3 large shallots, finely chopped
3 sprigs thyme, leaves only
30ml/2 tbsp finely chopped fresh tarragon
400g/14oz vegan 'chicken' pieces (e.g. Quorn/Gardein)
30ml/2 tbsp plain (all-purpose) flour, plus extra for dusting
175ml/6fl oz/¾ cup unsweetened soya milk
120ml/4fl oz/½ cup vegetable stock
7.5ml/1½ tsp fine salt
2.5ml/½ tsp ground black pepper
350g/12oz ready-made vegan puff pastry
green salad, or chips (fries) and peas, to serve

For the pastry glaze:
15ml/1 tbsp unsweetened soya milk
5ml/1 tsp maple syrup or golden syrup

1 Preheat the oven to 200°C/400°F/Gas 6. Put a baking sheet in the oven while it preheats. Grease the pie dish very well with oil.

2 Heat the oil in a large, wide pan or casserole, then add the mushrooms and fry over a medium heat for 10 minutes, stirring frequently, until softened. Add the chopped carrot, shallots, thyme and tarragon and cook for 10 more minutes.

3 Mix the vegan 'chicken' pieces into the mushroom mixture. Sprinkle over the flour and cook for 2 minutes, stirring.

4 Add half the soya milk and vegetable stock, stirring. Slowly bring to a boil, then add the rest of the milk and stock and bring back to a boil. Reduce the heat and simmer for a further 5 minutes. You should have a thick sauce.

5 Stir the salt and ground black pepper into the sauce and pour the mixture into the pie dish. The filling can mound, but don't fill so much that you think it's going to spill out. Set aside to cool completely, otherwise the pastry will be soggy underneath when cooked.

6 Sprinkle flour on a kitchen work surface and a rolling pin. Roll the pastry to 5mm/¼in thick to make the lid, using the dish as your guide for size.

7 Place the pastry lid over the filled pie and press the edges down to seal. Decorate by scoring the pastry lightly with a sharp knife in a trellis pattern. Be careful not to score right through the pastry. Poke a few small holes in the lid for the steam to escape.

8 Whisk the soya milk and syrup together in a small bowl and brush the glaze over the top of the pie, this gives a lovely golden finish. Put the pie on the preheated baking sheet to catch any overspill, then bake for 25–40 minutes until the pastry is golden brown and has puffed up.

9 Remove the pie from the oven and leave it to stand for 10 minutes before serving with a green salad, or traditional chips and peas.

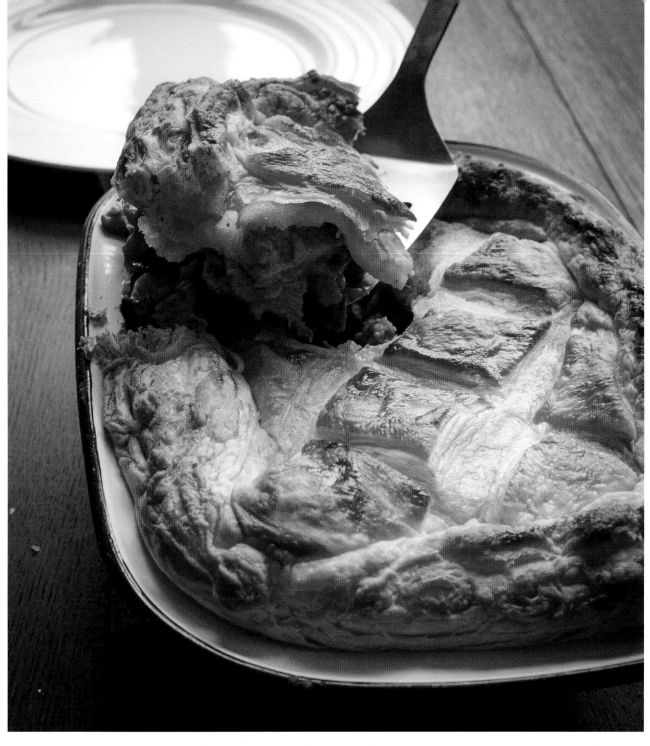

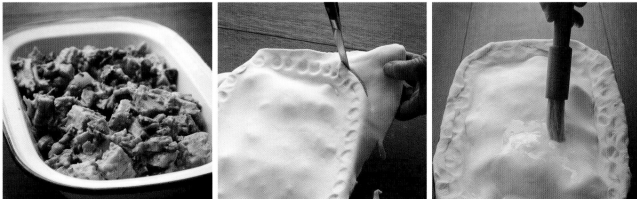

BOMBAY VEGETABLE PIE

I support Fulham Football Club. When I tried to recreate and 'veganise' their Bombay vegetable pie I was surprised that the only hits online when I searched for recipes were from 'thepiepundit' – a guy who goes round ranking the pies at various grounds – who remarked: 'not even this delicious specimen of a pie could mask the horrors of Fulham's performance, truly truly abysmal'. Hopefully my pie will bring a little more cheer to the table.

Serves: 6
Equipment: baking sheet, 25cm/10in-diameter pie dish, large, wide pan or casserole, rolling pin, whisk, small bowl, pastry brush
Prep time: 30 minutes, plus cooling
Cooking time: 1 hour 20 minutes

60ml/4 tbsp neutral vegetable oil, plus extra for greasing
1 large onion, finely chopped
3 large garlic cloves, finely chopped
2.5cm/1in piece of fresh root ginger, finely chopped
5ml/1 tsp ground coriander
5ml/1 tsp ground cumin
2.5ml/½ tsp ground turmeric
1.25ml/¼ tsp chilli powder
400g/14oz waxy potatoes, chopped into large dice
2 large carrots, diced
115g/4oz/1 cup frozen peas, thawed
45ml/3 tbsp plain (all-purpose) flour, plus extra for dusting
400ml/14fl oz/1⅔ cups unsweetened soya milk
5ml/1 tsp garam masala
6.25/1¼ tsp fine salt
500g/1¼lb ready-made vegan puff pastry

For the pastry glaze:
15ml/1 tbsp unsweetened soya milk
5ml/1 tsp maple syrup

1 Preheat the oven to 180°C/350°F/Gas 4. Put a baking sheet in the oven as it preheats. Grease the pie dish very well with oil.

2 Heat the oil in a large, wide pan or casserole, then add the onion, garlic and ginger and fry over a medium heat for 10 minutes, stirring frequently, until softened.

3 Stir in the ground coriander, cumin, turmeric and chilli powder and cook for 5 more minutes.

4 Stir in the potatoes and carrots and cook for 8 more minutes, stirring occasionally. Mix in the peas and cook for 2 minutes.

5 Sprinkle in the flour and cook for 2 minutes, stirring. Stir in half the soya milk. Bring to a boil, stirring, then lower the heat and simmer for a few minutes to cook the flour.

6 Add the remaining milk, bring to a boil, then reduce the heat and simmer for a few more minutes, until you have a thick sauce. Stir in the garam masala and salt and set aside to cool.

7 Sprinkle flour on a kitchen work surface and a rolling pin. Roll out two-thirds of the pastry to 5mm/¼in thick and use it to line the greased pie dish. Trim the edges and use the trimmings to patch any breaks or holes in the pastry. Roll out the remaining pastry to make the lid, using the dish as your guide for size. Set aside.

8 Spoon the curried vegetables into the pastry-lined pie dish. The filling can mound, but don't fill it so much that you think it's going to spill out.

9 Moisten the pastry rim with a little water, place the pastry lid on top and press the edges down to seal. Trim the edges with a knife, using the trimmings to make pastry leaves, if you fancy something fancy.

10 Whisk the soya milk and syrup together in a small bowl and brush all over the pastry lid. Poke a few small holes in the lid for the steam to escape.

11 Put the pie on the preheated baking sheet to catch any overspill, then bake for 45 minutes, until golden brown. Cover loosely with foil if the top starts to burn. Tuck in.

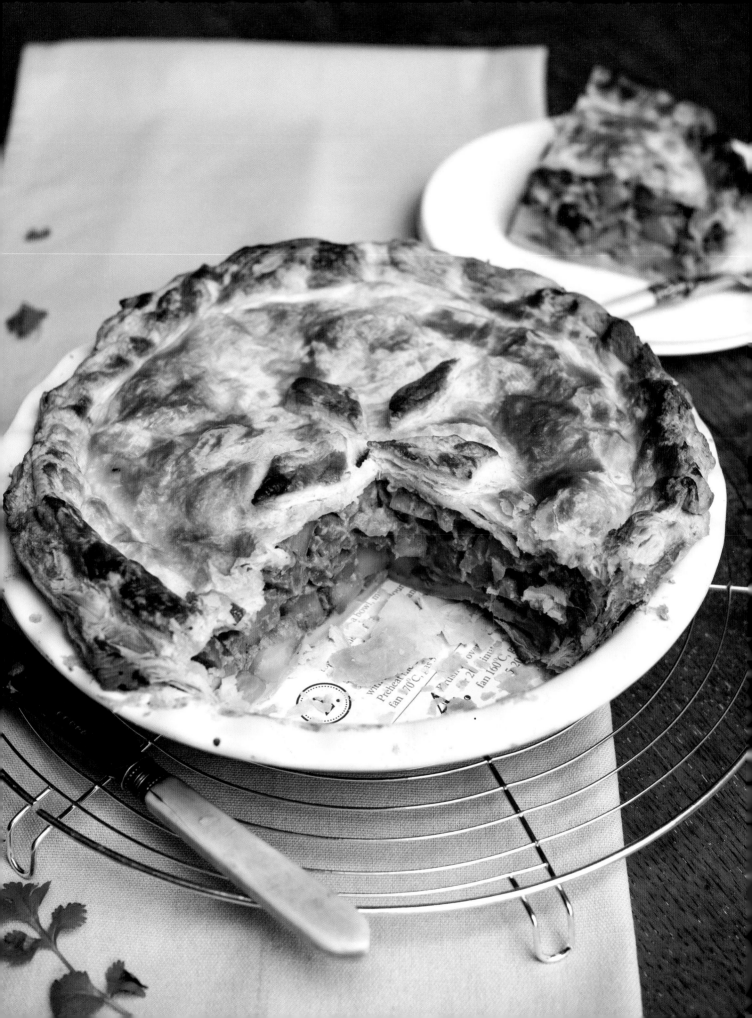

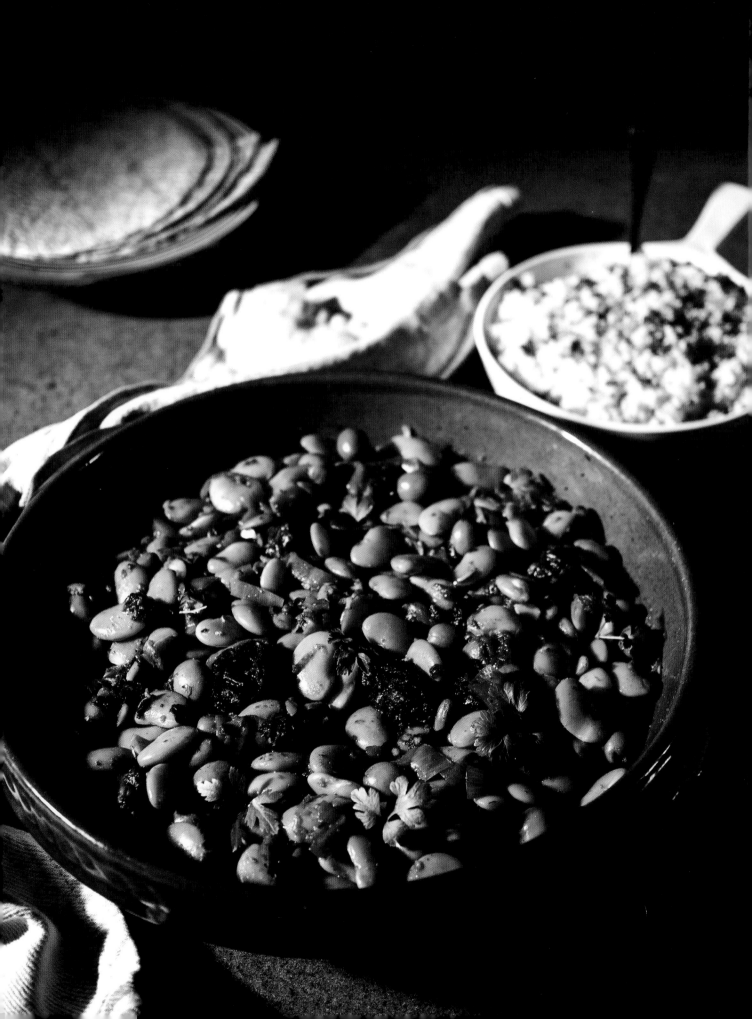

TAGINE OF BUTTER BEANS, OLIVES & PRUNES

Tagines have a distinctive flavour, mostly coming from sweet-and-sour combinations and liberal amounts of fresh parsley. Here, there is sweetness from prunes, cinnamon and ground ginger and sharpness from tart green olives. These contrasting flavours go perfectly with fat, creamy butter beans and fluffy couscous to soak up the juices.

Serves: 4
Equipment: large pan or casserole
Prep time: 20 minutes
Cooking time: 55 minutes

2 medium onions, thickly sliced
1 large carrot, chopped
1 large courgette (zucchini), chopped
2 garlic cloves, crushed
5ml/1 tsp ground cinnamon
5ml/1 tsp ground ginger
320g/11½oz/2 cups dried pitted prunes
175g/6oz/1½ cups stoned (pitted) green olives in brine (drained weight)
75g/3oz/½ cup blanched almonds
10 medium (about 5g/⅛oz) dried porcini mushrooms pieces
3 x 400g/14oz cans butter (lima) beans, drained
30ml/2 tbsp white wine vinegar
15ml/1 tbsp pomegranate molasses (optional)
5ml/1 tsp fine salt
2.5ml/½ tsp ground black pepper
300g/11oz/1¾ cups quick-cook couscous
60ml/4 tbsp finely chopped fresh parsley

SUBSTITUTE INGREDIENTS

Pitted prunes: *dried apricots*
Butter beans: *cannellini beans*
Pomegranate molasses: *golden (light corn) or agave syrup*
Couscous: *white or brown rice*

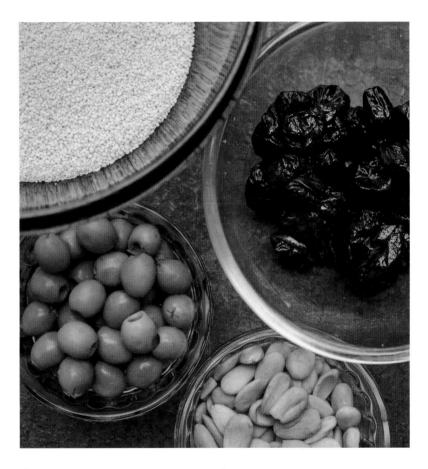

1 Put the onions, carrot, courgette, garlic, cinnamon, ginger, prunes, olives, almonds and mushrooms into a large pan or casserole. Pour in 1 litre/1¾ pints/4 cups water and gently mix around the ingredients. Bring to a boil, then reduce the heat to medium-low, cover and simmer gently for 45 minutes.

2 Stir in the butter beans, vinegar, pomegranate molasses (if using), salt and ground black pepper and simmer for 10 more minutes. If it looks like there isn't enough liquid, add a little more water.

3 Just after you've added the beans, cook the couscous according to the packet instructions.

4 Fluff the couscous with a fork and serve into wide bowls. Ladle on some of the tagine with some chopped parsley scattered on top.

THAI GREEN CURRY

When my good friend returned from Thailand, he handed me a scruffy, weathered recipe booklet held together by string – a truly authentic cookbook he'd been given at a local cooking class. I was intrigued by some of the techniques that were included, such as heating the coconut milk first so that it splits, and then using the separated coconut oil to fry the main ingredients – which, I discovered on further research, is the hallmark of a well-made Thai green curry. So here it is, in smartened-up and entirely vegan form.

Serves: 4
Equipment: kitchen paper or clean dish towels, heavy weight, medium baking tray, large pan or casserole
Prep time: 15 minutes, plus 30 minutes pressing
Cooking time: 30 minutes

400g/14oz extra-firm tofu, drained
2 large aubergines (eggplants), cut into 2.5cm/1in cubes
30ml/2 tbsp neutral vegetable oil
400ml/14oz can full-fat coconut milk (ideally around 18 per cent fat)
15–30ml/1–2 tbsp vegan Thai green curry paste*
4 fresh lime leaves, torn (optional) or 15ml/1 tbsp lime juice
225g/8oz sugar snap peas
5ml/1 tsp palm sugar or soft light brown sugar
10ml/2 tsp soy sauce
Perfect Basmati Rice (see page 61), to serve

* Check carefully that the curry paste is vegan, since traditional ones are not.

1 Preheat the oven to 180°C/350°F/Gas 4. Place several layers of kitchen paper, or a couple of clean dish towels, on a plate.

2 Put the tofu on the towels and cover with more paper/dish towels. Place a heavy object, such as a book or a heavy pan, on top to press the water out of the tofu. Leave to drain for at least 30 minutes. If you're short of time, press down on the heavy object to get as much water out of the tofu as possible. Slice into 2.5cm/1in cubes.

3 Toss the aubergines with the oil on a medium baking tray and roast in the oven for 15–20 minutes, until the aubergine is golden brown and softened but not mushy.

4 Meanwhile, scoop 60ml/4 tbsp of the coconut cream from the top of the coconut milk can into a large pan or casserole and place over a medium heat. After about 5 minutes (sometimes a little longer) the coconut cream should split into oil and coconut solids. If the coconut milk you're using has been homogenised, do this step anyway, though the coconut milk won't split.

5 Stir the Thai green curry paste into the split coconut milk. If you're sensitive to spice, only use 15ml/1 tbsp. Sauté for 2 minutes.

6 Gently mix in the cubed tofu and sauté over a medium-high heat for 10 minutes.

7 Add 175ml/6fl oz/¾ cup water, the roasted aubergine, kaffir lime leaves, if using, and the rest of the coconut milk. Bring to a boil, then reduce the heat and simmer for 10 minutes so the liquid reduces. Add the sugar snap peas for the last 3 minutes of the cooking time.

8 Stir in the sugar and soy sauce. If you're not using the kaffir lime leaves, add the lime juice now. Serve with rice.

SUBSTITUTE INGREDIENTS
Fresh kaffir lime leaves: *dried lime leaves*
Palm sugar: *dark soft brown sugar*
Soy sauce: *tamari sauce*

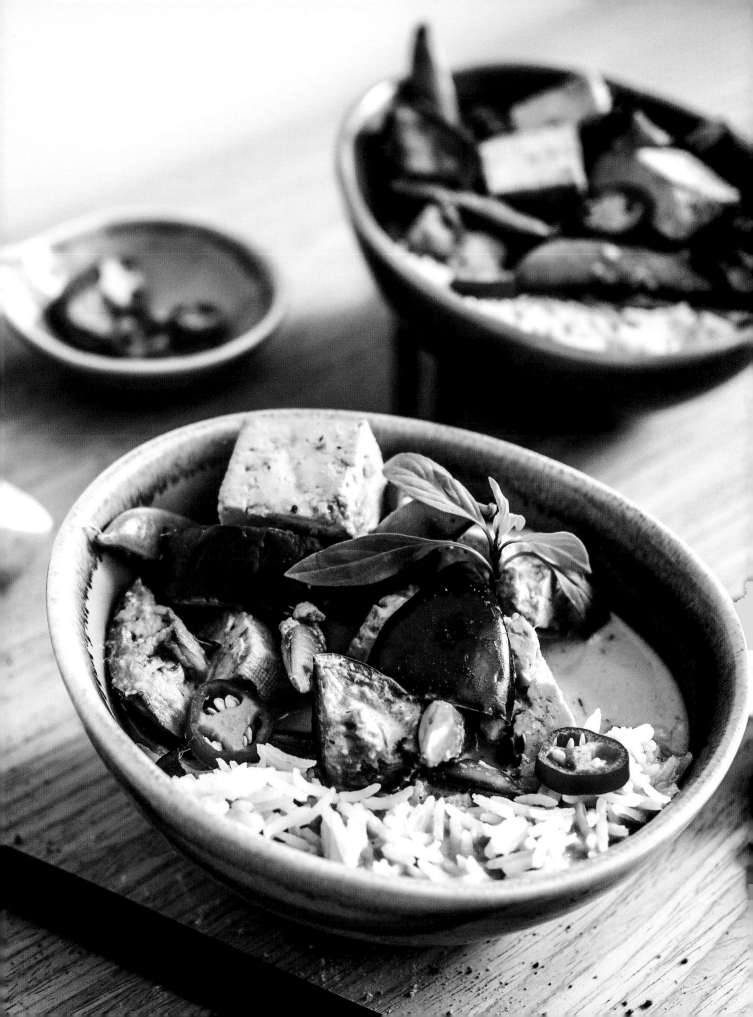

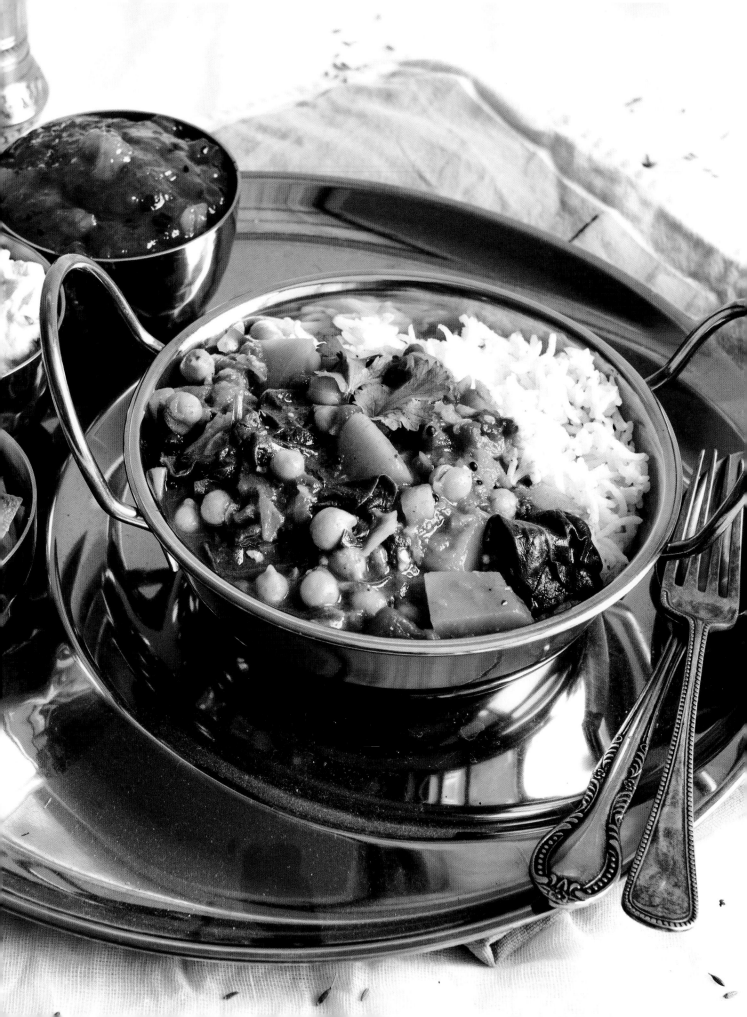

CHICKPEA, BUTTERNUT SQUASH & SPINACH CURRY

Serves: 4–6
Equipment: large pan or casserole
Prep time: 15 minutes
Cooking time: about 45 minutes

If you have canned tomatoes, pulses and coconut milk, plus some standard spices, stocked in the cupboard, you'll always be able to whip up this delicious one-pot curry at a moment's notice. It's very cheap, too.

60ml/4 tbsp neutral vegetable oil

5ml/1 tsp black mustard seeds

2 medium onions, finely chopped

6 garlic cloves, finely chopped

5cm/2in piece of fresh root ginger, finely chopped

15ml/1 tbsp tomato paste

7.5ml/1½ tsp ground cumin

7.5ml/1½ tsp ground coriander

5ml/1 tsp ground turmeric

2.5ml/½ tsp chilli powder

1 large butternut squash, peeled, seeded and chopped into 2.5cm/1in cubes

400g/14oz can chopped tomatoes

400g/14oz can full-fat coconut milk

7.5ml/1½ tsp fine salt

3.75ml/¾ tsp sugar

7.5ml/1½ tsp garam masala

2 x 400g/14oz cans chickpeas, drained

250g/9oz baby spinach

a packed handful (about 15g/½oz) of fresh coriander (cilantro), roughly chopped

Perfect Basmati Rice (see page 61), fresh lime wedges and mango chutney, to serve

1 Heat the oil in a large pan or casserole over a high heat. Add the mustard seeds and fry for 30–60 seconds, until they start to pop.

2 Turn the heat down to medium and add the onion. Cook for 5 minutes.

3 Add the garlic, ginger and tomato paste and cook for 5 more minutes, then stir in the spices and cook for 5 more minutes.

4 Add the butternut squash, coating it in the onion mixture, then add the chopped tomatoes, coconut milk and 250ml/8fl oz/1 cup water. Bring to a boil, then turn down the heat and simmer for 25 minutes or until the squash is soft.

5 Stir in the salt, sugar and garam masala, followed by the chickpeas and spinach. Cook for about 5 more minutes, until the spinach wilts.

6 Sprinkle over the fresh coriander and serve with rice, lime wedges and mango chutney.

SUBSTITUTE INGREDIENTS
Black mustard seeds: *cumin seeds*
Canned tomatoes: *fresh tomatoes*
Baby spinach: *spring greens or kale*

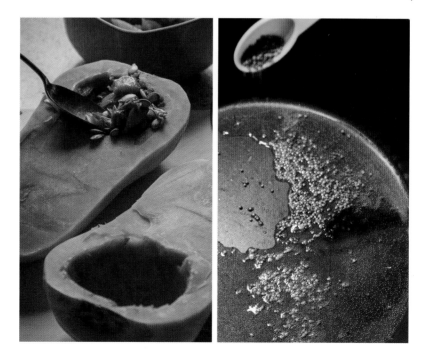

WEST AFRICAN PEANUT STEW

I love the North and West African tradition of using sweet, warm spices with savoury ingredients. Here, cardamom, cinnamon, cloves and ground ginger are paired with aubergine and okra in a spicy peanut sauce. This stew only improves with age (don't we all), so it's worth making double and freezing half.

Serves: 4
Equipment: large pan or casserole or 2 large pans
Prep time: 20 minutes
Cooking time: 55 minutes

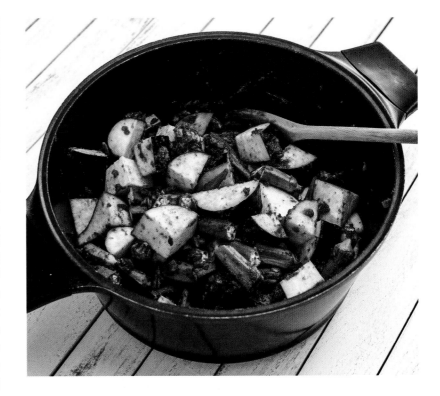

45ml/3 tbsp neutral vegetable oil
1 large onion, finely chopped
2.5cm/1in piece of fresh root ginger, finely chopped
1 fresh red chilli, seeded and finely chopped
2.5ml/½ tsp ground cumin
2.5ml/½ tsp ground coriander
2.5ml/½ tsp cinnamon
1.25ml/¼ tsp ground ginger
2.5ml/½ tsp ground black pepper
1 cardamom pod, seeds only, crushed
1.25ml/¼ tsp ground cloves
22.5ml/1½ tbsp tomato paste
90ml/6 tbsp smooth peanut butter
2 large aubergines (eggplants), chopped into 2.5cm/1in chunks
350g/12oz fresh okra, roughly chopped
2 large ripe tomatoes, roughly chopped
300g/11oz/1½ cups brown rice
2.5ml/½ tsp sugar
5ml/1 tsp fine salt
15ml/1 tbsp lime juice
30ml/2 tbsp finely chopped fresh parsley

1 Heat the oil in a large pan or casserole over a medium heat. Add the onion and sauté for 15 minutes, adding the ginger and chilli after 10 minutes. Stir all the spices into the onion mixture, and cook for 5 more minutes.

2 Add the tomato paste and peanut butter and stir to combine well. Cook for 3 more minutes.

3 Stir in the aubergine and okra so it is well coated, then add the tomatoes and 750ml/1¼ pints/3 cups water, stir, and bring to a boil. Reduce the heat and simmer for 25 minutes, until thick.

4 Meanwhile, bring 1 litre/1¾ pints/4 cups water to a boil in a large pan. Add the brown rice, lower the heat to a simmer and cook according to packet instructions or until tender. Drain well.

5 Stir the sugar, salt and lime juice into the peanut stew, sprinkle over the parsley and serve with the rice.

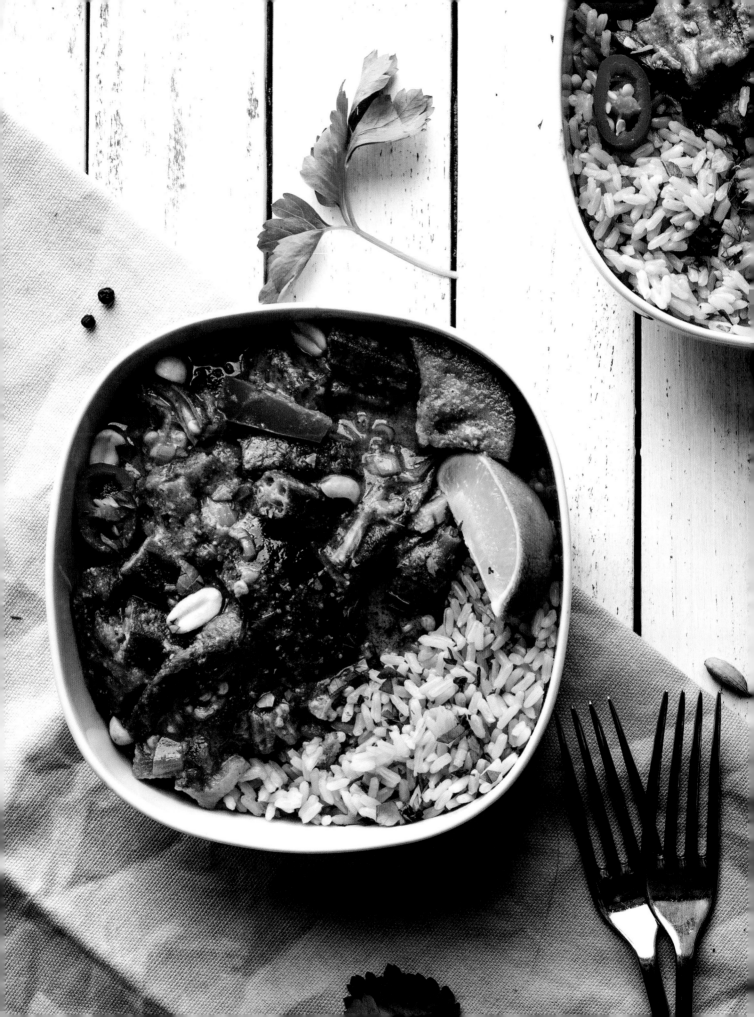

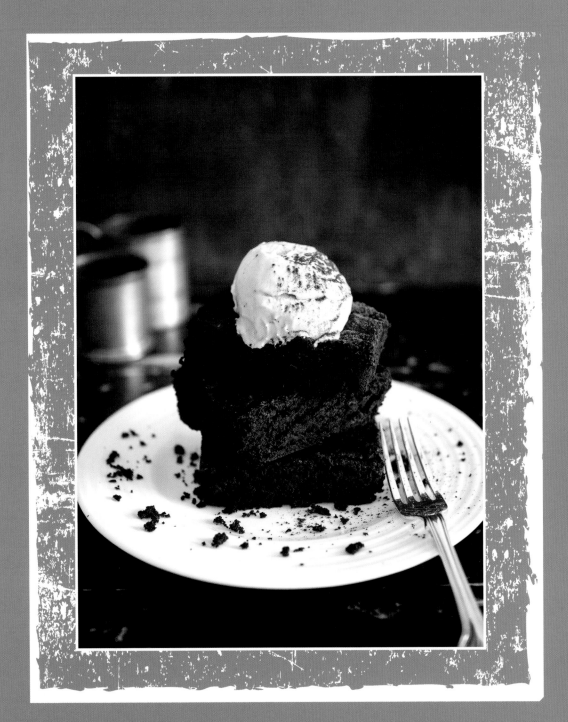

DESSERTS, SWEET TREATS AND BREADS

HAZELNUT RICE PUDDING

This is my mum's desert island dessert. She says the world divides into two types of people: those who like rice pudding with a skin and those who don't. I'm in the latter camp. She recently discovered hazelnut milk, which makes rice pudding absurdly delicious and removes the need for added sugar.

Serves: 4
Equipment: roughly 30 x 20cm/12 x 8in ovenproof dish
Prep time: 1 minute
Cooking time: 60–90 minutes

1 Preheat the oven to 160°C/325°F/Gas 3. Mix the rice and plant-based milks in the ovenproof dish, then bake for 60–90 minutes, depending on the preferred consistency.

2 If you like the skin, don't stir during the cooking time, but watch the pudding – you might need to pierce the skin to let the steam escape. If you don't want a skin to form, stir every 15–20 minutes.

3 Allow the pudding to stand for a few minutes, then serve with the fruit.

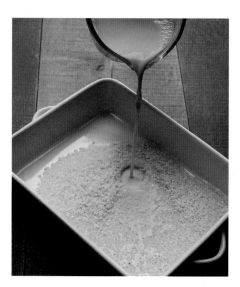

100g/3½oz/½ cups pudding rice
500ml/17fl oz/generous 2 cups sweetened hazelnut milk
500ml/17fl oz/generous 2 cups sweetened hemp milk
fruit compote, to serve

SUBSTITUTE INGREDIENTS
Any plant-based milk can be used instead of hazelnut or hemp milk. If using unsweetened milks add 15–30ml/1–2 tbsp sugar for each milk to the mixture before baking.

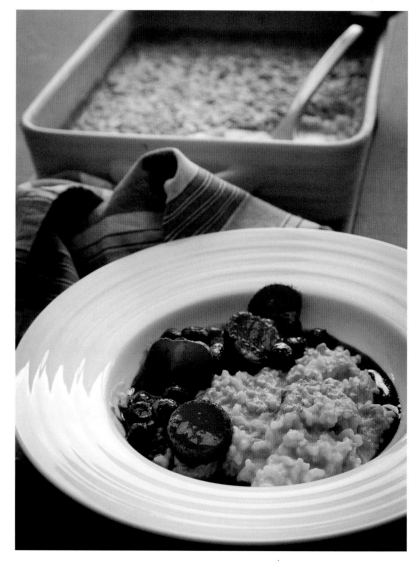

MIXED BERRY CRUMBLE

You could easily make a crumble topping out of just flour, fat and sugar. However, I like to enhance mine by adding ground almonds instead of some of the flour, rolled oats for their wholesomeness and visual contrast, and buckwheat groats for their nubbly texture and nutty flavour.

Serves: 4–6
Equipment: food processor or large bowl, 28 x 23 x 5cm/11 x 9 x 2in ovenproof baking dish, baking tray, foil
Prep time: 10 minutes
Cooking time: 40–50 minutes

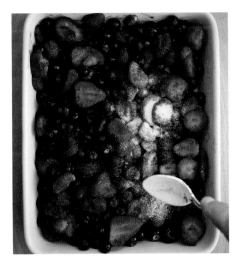

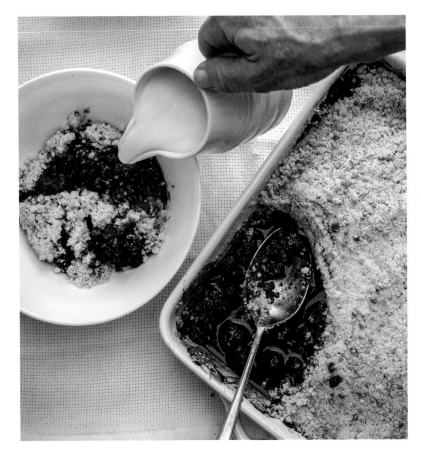

190g/6½oz/1⅔ cups plain (all-purpose) flour

175g/6oz/1½ cups ground almonds

1.25ml/¼ tsp fine salt

150g/5oz/10 tbsp cold baking block margarine, cubed

50g/2oz/½ cup rolled oats

90g/3½oz/½ cup caster (superfine) sugar

65g/2½oz/⅓ cup buckwheat groats

1.2kg/2½lb mixed frozen fruit, such as raspberries, blackberries or blackcurrants

about 30ml/2 tbsp caster (superfine) sugar

vegan ice cream, custard or cream, to serve

1 Put the flour, ground almonds, salt and cubed margarine into a food processor. Pulse until the mixture resembles large breadcrumbs but stop before it clumps together. If you don't have a food processor, rub the butter into the flour and ground almonds with your fingers in a large bowl.

2 Preheat the oven to 180°C/350°F/Gas 4. Add the oats to the food processor and pulse a couple times, or stir the oats into the flour mixture in the bowl. Stir in the sugar and buckwheat groats.

3 Put the mixed fruit in the baking dish and sprinkle over the sugar. You may want to add a little more, depending on what type of fruit you use. Sprinkle the topping mixture evenly on top of the fruit.

4 Put the crumble on a baking tray to catch any spills, then bake for about 40–50 minutes, until golden brown. Remove from the oven and allow to cool for at least 10 minutes. Serve with vegan ice cream, custard or cream.

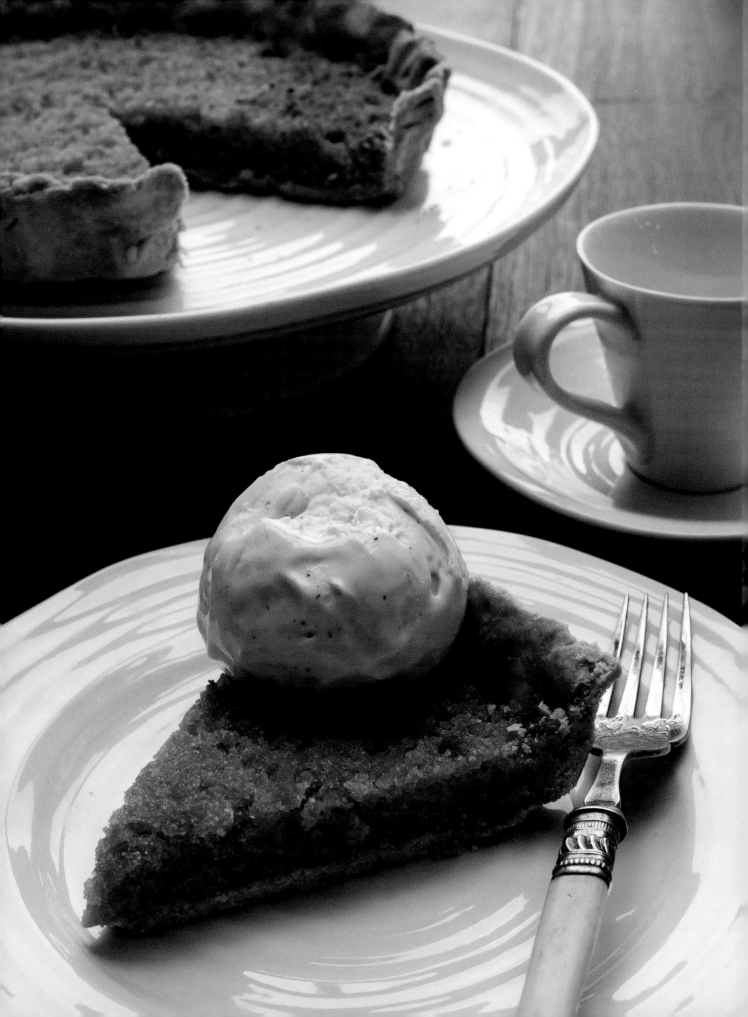

TREACLE TART

Treacle tart is one of those desserts where substitutions won't really work. Old-fashioned golden syrup and white breadcrumbs, after a spell in the oven, have a uniquely sticky, granular, just-set consistency that enables you to eat far more golden syrup than is sensible. In a good way.

Serves: 8
Equipment: food processor or large bowl, clear film (plastic wrap), 23cm/9in loose-bottomed tart tin (pan), fork, medium baking tray, baking parchment, ceramic baking beans, uncooked rice or dried pulses, medium bowl, foil
Prep time: 25 minutes, plus 1 hour chilling
Cooking time: 50 minutes

For the pastry:
225g/8oz/2 cups plain (all-purpose) flour, plus extra for dusting
115g/4oz/½ cup cold baking block margarine, cubed, plus extra for greasing
5ml/1 tsp caster (superfine) sugar
0.6ml/⅛ tsp salt

For the filling:
450g/1lb/1⅓ cups golden (light corn) syrup
150g/5oz/3 cups fresh white breadcrumbs
30ml/2 tbsp lemon juice
vegan ice cream, cream or custard, to serve

1 To make the pastry, put the flour, margarine, sugar and salt in a food processor (if you don't have one, see step 2). Pulse about 10 times to mix the ingredients together. Add 60ml/4 tbsp cold water to the food processor and pulse about 10 more times until the mixture comes together.

2 To make the pastry by hand, put all the ingredients into a large bowl. Rub the margarine, sugar and salt into the flour with your fingertips until the mixture resembles breadcrumbs. Add 60ml/4 tbsp cold water gradually until the pastry comes together into a ball.

3 Wrap the pastry in clear film and chill in the fridge for 30 minutes. Grease the tart tin.

4 Sprinkle a little flour on a kitchen work surface. Roll the pastry out to 5mm/¼in thick.

5 Use the rolled pastry to line the tart tin. Prick the bottom a few times with a fork. Chill for a further 30 minutes in the fridge.

6 Preheat the oven to 180°C/350°F/Gas 4. Place a medium baking tray in the oven.

7 To blind bake the pastry, loosely cover the pastry-lined tin with a large piece of baking parchment. Put a handful of ceramic baking beans, uncooked rice or dried pulses on to the baking parchment to weight it down. Bake for 15 minutes, then remove the paper and weights and bake for 5 minutes more.

8 Meanwhile, make the filling by measuring the golden syrup into a medium bowl and mixing in the breadcrumbs and lemon juice.

9 Remove the pastry case from the oven and fill it with the golden syrup and breadcrumb mixture.

10 Return to the oven and bake for 30 minutes, checking regularly. If the top is starting to burn, cover loosely with foil.

11 Leave to cool for at least 15 minutes before serving. Serve with vegan ice cream, cream or custard.

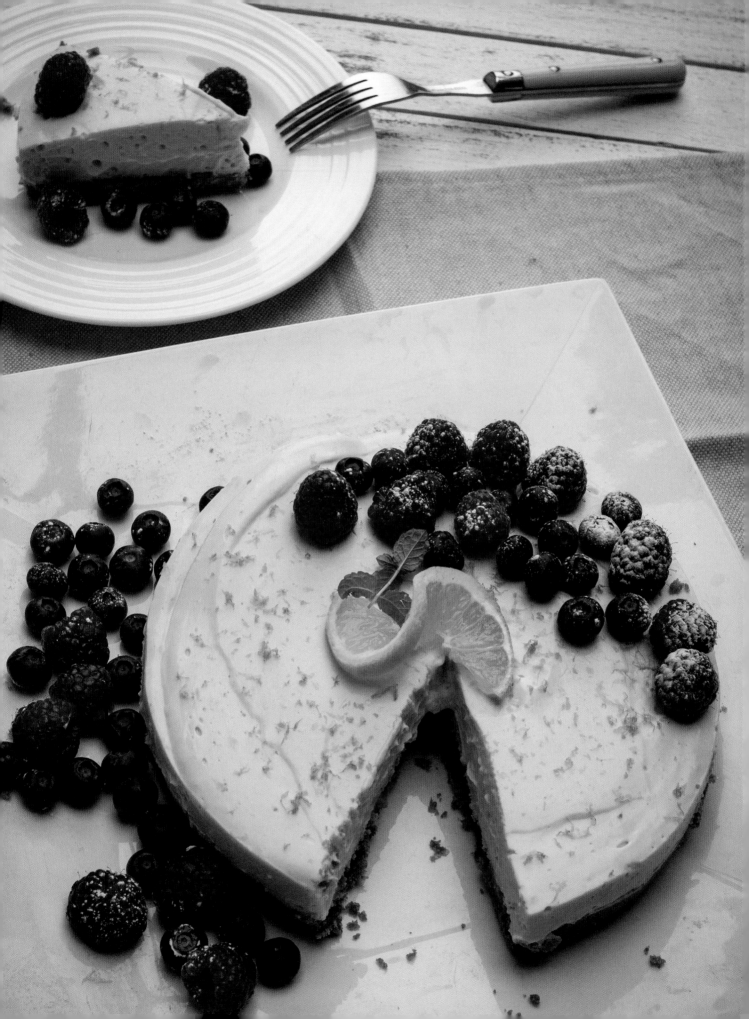

LEMON NO-BAKE CHEESECAKE

This recipe is a great example of how clever vegan substitutes can reopen the door to a classic dessert that most would imagine unadaptable for vegans: block margarine in the crumbly biscuit base, and coconut cream in the thick, rich topping. Served with some fresh summer berries, this is a classic dessert that will wow all your guests, whether vegan or not.

Serves: 8
Equipment: 20cm/8in springform or loose-bottomed cake tin (pan), baking parchment, heatproof bowl, food processor or strong plastic bag and rolling pin, medium pan, small bowl, whisk, jug blender or bowl and stick blender, spatula
Prep time: 30 minutes, plus at least 4 hours chilling
Cooking time: 5 minutes

For the biscuit base:
75g/3oz/6 tbsp baking block margarine, plus extra for greasing
150g/5oz vegan digestive biscuits (graham crackers)
100g/3¾oz ginger nut biscuits (ginger snaps)

For the lemon cheesecake topping:
200g/7oz/scant 1 cup coconut cream
175ml/6fl oz/¾ cup lemon juice (juice of about 6 medium lemons)
zest of 2 medium lemons
50g/2oz/¼ cup caster (superfine) sugar
45g/1⅔oz/3 tbsp baking block margarine
25g/1oz/¼ cup cornflour (corn starch)
300g/11oz/1¼ cups silken tofu
115g/4oz/½ cup vegan cream cheese (e.g. Tofutti, or supermarket own brand)

For the topping (suggestions):
fresh berries or chopped nuts, sprigs of fresh mint and lemon zest, icing (confectioners') sugar, for dusting

1 Grease the cake tin well with a little margarine. Line the base of the tin with baking parchment.

2 For the biscuit base, melt the block margarine in a heatproof bowl in the microwave on low (it will only take 20–30 seconds).

3 Put the digestive and ginger biscuits in a food processor and pulse about 10 times to a fine breadcrumb consistency. Alternatively, put the biscuits in a strong plastic bag, seal it and bash them with a rolling pin.

4 Add the melted margarine to the food processor and pulse a few times to mix it in, or add the crushed biscuits to the bowl in which the butter was melted, and stir to combine.

5 Transfer the base mixture to the greased cake tin. Press down with your hands to create a compressed, even layer. Chill in the fridge while you make the topping.

6 For the lemon topping, put all the ingredients except for the cornflour, tofu and cream cheese in a medium pan over a low heat. Slowly bring the mixture to a gentle simmer, stirring.

7 Remove the pan from the heat as soon as the ingredients have come together. Allow to cool for a few minutes.

8 Working quickly, whisk the cornflour with 45ml/3 tbsp water in a small bowl and add it to the warm coconut-lemon juice mixture, whisking constantly to prevent any lumps from forming. Allow to cool for another few minutes.

9 Blend the tofu and cream cheese very well in a food processor or jug blender, or in a bowl with a stick blender.

10 Add the lemon mixture to the tofu/cream cheese and whizz again until it is very smooth.

11 Pour the topping into the chilled biscuit base, smoothing and evening out the top with a spatula. Return to the fridge for at least 4 hours, or you can leave it overnight.

12 Carefully remove the cheesecake from the tin on to a serving plate. Sprinkle over fresh berries, chopped nuts or whichever topping you prefer.

PEANUT BUTTER CHOCOLATE CHIP COOKIES

Peanut butter chocolate chip cookies. I'm not sure I need to say anything else. Peanut butter. Chocolate chip. Cookies. If you object, consult a doctor. Or make something else.

Makes: 12–14 cookies
Equipment: large bowl, food processor, fork, 2 large or 3 medium baking trays, baking parchment, spatula or spoon (optional), small bowl, wire rack
Prep time: 15 minutes, plus 15 minutes soaking
Cooking time: 15–25 minutes

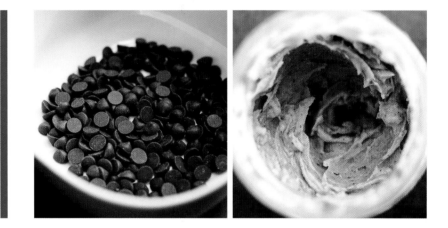

30ml/2 tbsp ground flaxseeds/linseeds
90g/3½oz/1 cup rolled oats
130g/4½oz/generous 1 cup plain (all-purpose) flour
5ml/1 tsp baking powder
130g/4½oz/⅔ cup caster (superfine) sugar
0.6ml/⅛ tsp fine salt
150g/9oz/⅔ cup creamy smooth peanut butter*
90ml/6 tbsp unsweetened plant-based milk
30g/1½oz/scant ¼ cup vegan dark (bittersweet) chocolate chips

If you're using unsweetened, unsalted peanut butter, add an extra 0.6ml/⅛ tsp sugar and 0.6ml/⅛ tsp salt.

SUBSTITUTE INGREDIENTS
Flaxseeds/linseeds: *1 large ripe banana, mashed. Add more banana if the mixture isn't holding together by the end of step 3.*

1 Mix the ground flaxseeds or linseeds with 75ml/5 tbsp water in a large bowl. Set aside to soak for 15 minutes for the gel to thicken. Preheat the oven to 180°C/350°F/Gas 4.

2 Put the oats, flour, baking powder, sugar and salt in a food processor and blitz for about 15 seconds.

3 Mix the peanut butter and plant-based milk into the flaxseed/linseed gel as well as you can with a fork. Add this to the food processor and pulse until combined into a sticky ball. Avoid overmixing.

4 Line 2 large or 3 medium baking trays with baking parchment and scoop out the mixture into the large bowl from before. Wet your hands, or use a damp spatula to mix half of the chocolate chips into the cookie mixture.

5 Fill a small bowl with water and set it next to the baking trays, so that while shaping the cookies you can periodically wet your hands so that the mixture doesn't stick to them.

6 Weigh out 50g/2oz pieces of cookie mixture and space out evenly on the baking trays. You should have enough to create 12–14 balls of dough. Flatten each ball into a 1cm/½in-high cookie shape with the flats of your fingers. Push the remaining chocolate chips into the surface of the cookies.

7 Bake for 15 minutes, rotating and swapping the trays around after 10 minutes to make sure they bake evenly. It's likely they will need 5 more minutes; just bake until nicely browned. Err on the side of under rather than overbaked. Leave to cool on the trays for 10 minutes, then carefully transfer to a wire rack to cool completely.

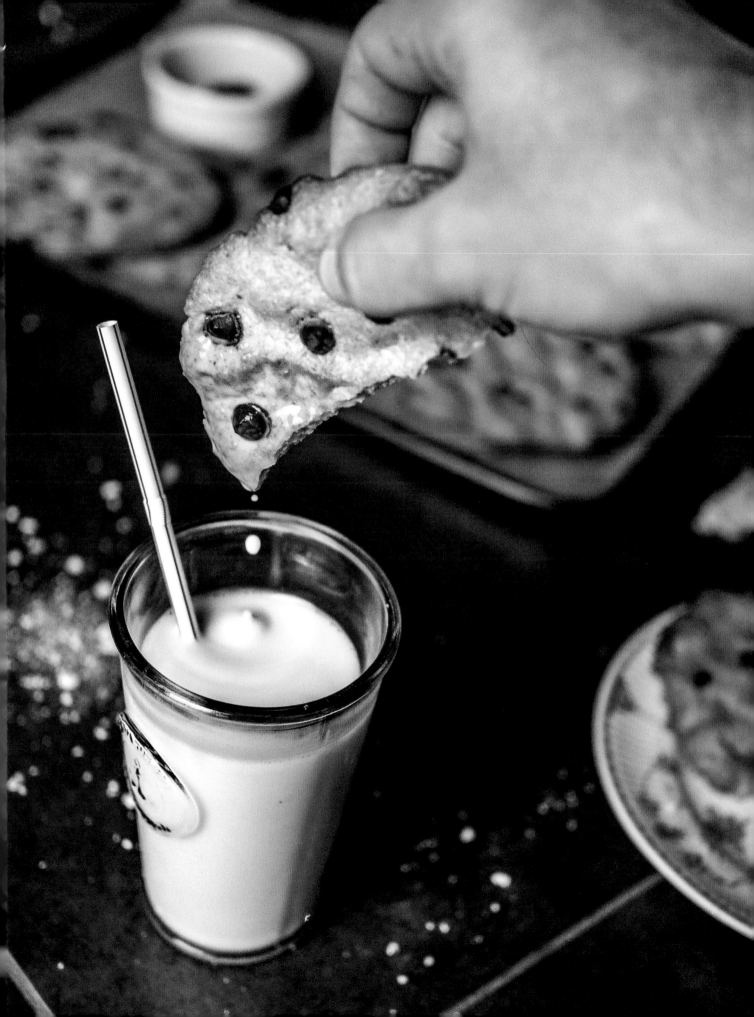

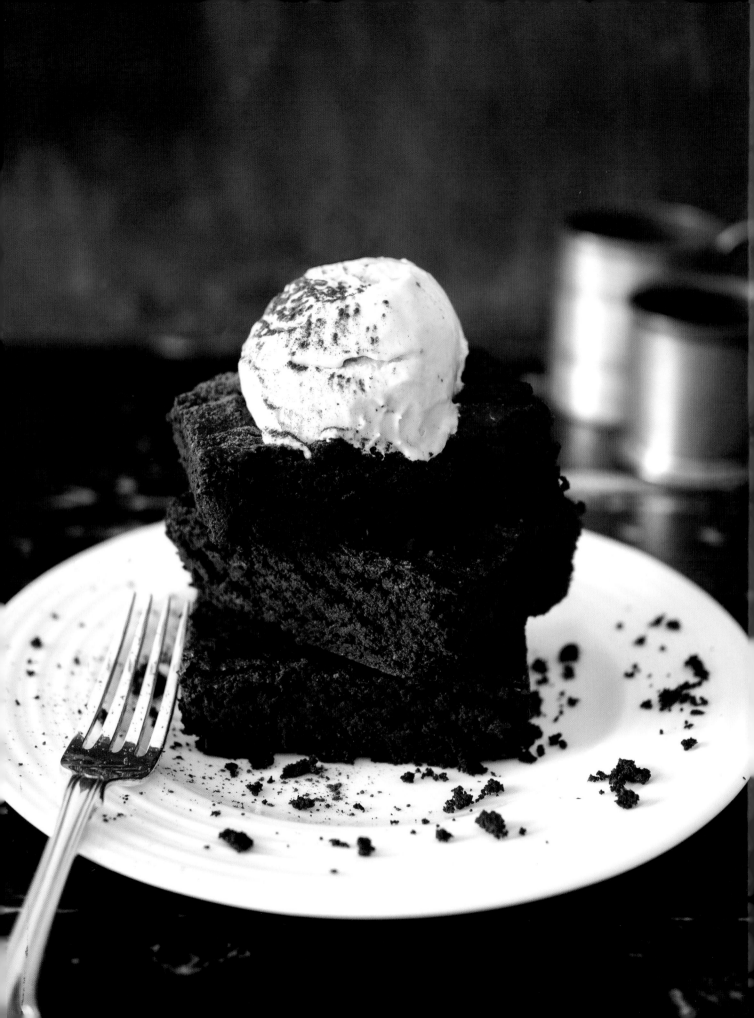

DOUBLE CHOCOLATE CHUNK BROWNIES

Many vegan cookbooks include a recipe for (in my opinion) rather worthy sweet potato brownies. Not here. These brownies are rich, dark and dense – perfect with a scoop of dairy-free ice cream, of which there are now many excellent and widely available vegan varieties.

Makes: 12 large or 16 small brownies
Equipment: 30 x 20 x 5cm/12 x 8 x 2in baking tray, baking parchment, small bowl, sieve (strainer), 1 or 2 heatproof bowls, small pan (optional), spatula, foil (optional)
Prep time: 20 minutes, plus 15 minutes soaking
Cooking time: 25 minutes

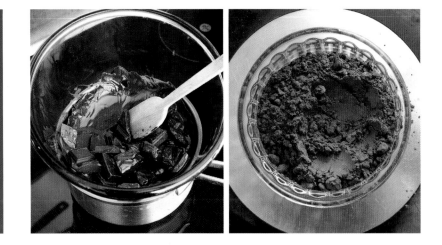

30ml/2 tbsp ground flaxseeds/linseeds
275g/10oz vegan dark (bittersweet) chocolate
90g/3½oz/¾ cup plain (all-purpose) flour
50g/2oz/½ cup unsweetened cocoa powder
7.5ml/1½ tsp baking powder
1.25ml/¼ tsp fine salt
200g/7oz/1 cup caster (superfine) sugar
150g/5oz/10 tbsp baking block margarine, plus extra for greasing
90ml/6 tbsp unsweetened plant-based milk

1 Mix the flaxseeds/linseeds with 90ml/6 tbsp water in a small bowl. Set aside to soak for 15 minutes to thicken into a gel. Preheat the oven to 180°C/350°F/Gas 4. Grease and line the baking tray.

2 Break off 75g/3oz of the dark chocolate and chop it into rough chunks. Set the remaining chocolate aside for later.

3 Sift the flour, cocoa powder, baking powder and salt into a large bowl. Stir in the sugar and chocolate chunks and set aside.

4 Melt the reserved 200g/7oz dark chocolate on low power in a heatproof bowl in the microwave or over a small pan of barely simmering water.

5 Once the chocolate has melted, either melt the margarine in another bowl in the microwave, or add the margarine to the heatproof bowl above the water and let that melt too. Remove from the heat.

6 Stir the flaxseed/linseed gel and the plant-based milk into the chocolate-margarine mixture. Mix the melted chocolate mixture into the dry ingredients using a spatula.

7 Pour the mixture into the lined baking tray and bake for 25 minutes, until just set but still with a bit of give in the centre. Keep an eye on it as it can burn easily, covering with foil if necessary.

8 Remove from the oven and leave to cool completely in the tray. Cut into 12 pieces for large brownies or 16 pieces for small ones.

CELEBRATION CHOCOLATE CAKE

A rich, indulgent cake with a hint of coffee, this is perfect for birthdays and celebrations. Somehow the cocoa powder removes the need for an egg substitute (I've tried to find out why, in vain!). If only cocoa powder were always suitable where eggs are used as a binder – vegan cocoa 'meatballs' anyone?

Makes: 1 large cake
Equipment: 20cm/8in-diameter springform cake tin (pan), baking parchment or cake liner, sieve (strainer), 2 large bowls, small bowl, medium pan, spatula or wooden spoon, foil, skewer, wire rack, electric whisk, foil (optional)
Prep time: 25 minutes, plus cooling
Cooking time: 45 minutes–1 hour

225g/8oz/2 cups plain (all-purpose) flour
75g/3oz/²⁄₃ cup unsweetened cocoa powder
15ml/1 tbsp baking powder
300g/11oz/1½ cups caster (superfine) sugar
1.25ml/¼ tsp fine salt
5ml/1 tsp instant coffee granules
150g/5oz/10 tbsp baking block margarine, plus extra for greasing
300ml/½ pint/1¼ cups unsweetened plant-based milk, e.g. soya

For the frosting:
75g/3oz/6 tbsp baking block margarine, at room temperature
200g/7oz/1¾ cup icing (confectioners') sugar
30ml/2 tbsp unsweetened cocoa powder

1 Preheat the oven to 170°C/340ºF/Gas 3½. Grease the cake tin with a little margarine, then line it with baking parchment. Sift the flour, cocoa powder and baking powder into a large bowl, then stir in the sugar and salt.

2 In a small bowl, dissolve the coffee granules in 10ml/2 tsp boiling water. Melt the margarine in a medium pan on the hob. Allow to cool for a couple of minutes, then stir in the plant-based milk and dissolved coffee granules.

3 Add the wet ingredients to the dry ones and mix together with a spatula or wooden spoon. Do not overmix; the mixture should be quite runny. Pour the batter into the lined cake tin and bake for 45 minutes. Check after 25 minutes; if the top is beginning to burn, cover loosely with foil.

4 Check the cake is done by inserting a skewer into the middle. It should come out clean. If it doesn't, bake for 10–15 more minutes.

5 Once done, leave the cake to cool in its tin for 10 minutes, then transfer to a wire rack and leave to cool completely.

6 For the frosting, put the margarine in a large bowl and sift over the icing sugar and cocoa powder. Beat well with an electric whisk until soft peaks are formed. If you don't have an electric whisk, beat the ingredients together vigorously with a wooden spoon. Add water 15ml/1 tbsp at a time if the mixture is too thick to spread.

7 Slice the cake in half horizontally with a sharp knife. Spread a thin layer of icing on the cut side of one of the cakes. Put the un-iced cake half back on top, then spread the remaining icing on top of the whole cake.

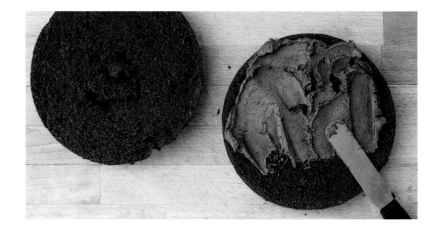

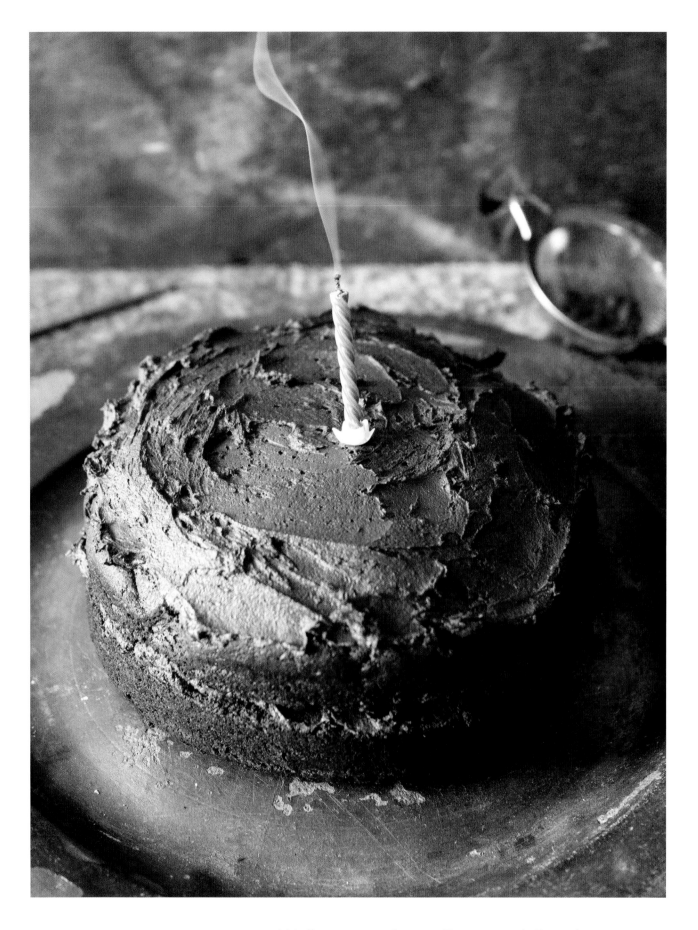

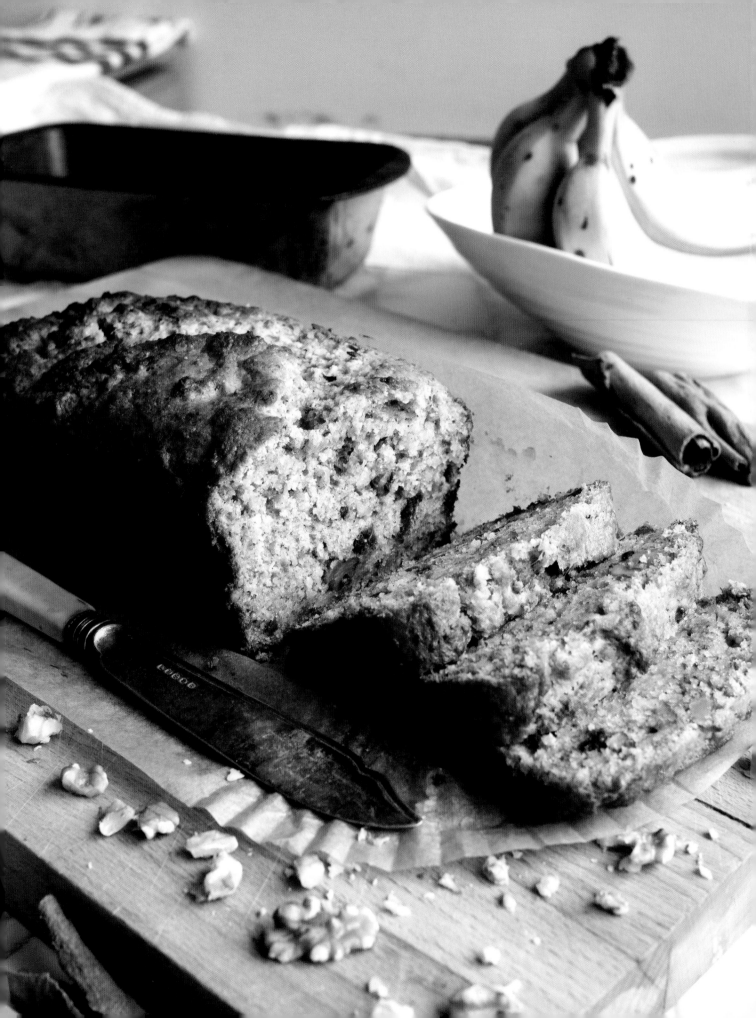

NUTTY BANANA BREAD

Banana bread is the perfect vegan bake because bananas act as a binder and eliminate the need for eggs to hold the risen cake together. This one has my favourite additions of walnuts and chopped dates, with a dash of ground ginger, cinnamon and nutmeg. Ground oats give the cake a crumbly texture and slightly more wholesome flavour.

Makes: 1 loaf
Equipment: 20 x 10 x 7.5cm/8 x 4 x 3in (900g/2lb) loaf tin (pan), food processor or blender, sieve (strainer), large bowl, heatproof bowl or small pan, foil, skewer, wire rack
Prep time: 15 minutes
Cooking time: 50–60 minutes

90g/3½oz/1 cup rolled oats

150g/5oz/1¼ cups plain (all-purpose) flour

15ml/1 tbsp baking powder

1.25ml/¼ tsp fine salt

90g/3½oz/½ cup caster (superfine) sugar

30g/1½oz/¼ cup roughly chopped walnuts

30g/1½oz/¼ cup chopped stoned (pitted) dates

2.5ml/½ tsp ground cinnamon

0.6ml/⅛ tsp ground nutmeg

1.25ml/¼ tsp ground ginger

115g/4oz/½ cup baking block margarine, plus extra for greasing

45ml/3 tbsp unsweetened plant-based milk

15ml/1 tbsp lemon juice

3 large or 4 medium very ripe bananas (total peeled weight 375g/13oz)

SUBSTITUTE INGREDIENTS
Walnuts: *hazelnuts*
Dates: *raisins, sultanas or chopped dried apricots*

1 Preheat the oven to 180°C/350°F/Gas 4. Grease the loaf tin with a little margarine and line with baking parchment.

2 Blitz the oats to a coarse flour in a food processor or blender.

3 Sift the flour, baking powder and salt into a large bowl, then mix in the oat flour, sugar, walnuts, dates and spices.

4 Gently melt the margarine in a heatproof bowl in the microwave or in a small pan over the hob, then combine with the plant-based milk and lemon juice. Mash the bananas into this mixture.

5 Add the banana mixture to the dry ingredients and mix just to combine. Do not overmix.

6 Spoon the mixture into the loaf tin and bake for 50 minutes. Cover loosely with foil if the top is beginning to burn.

7 Test to see the banana bread is cooked by inserting a skewer in the middle of the cake. If it comes out clean the banana bread is done. If not, bake for another 10 minutes or so.

8 Remove from the oven and leave to cool in the tin for 10 minutes, then transfer to a wire rack and leave to cool completely. It freezes well.

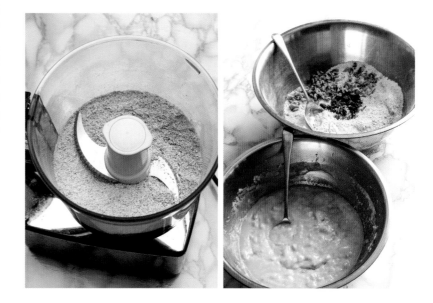

SPIRAL SEEDED PROTEIN BREAD

In this recipe, chia, flaxseeds and pumpkin seeds, wholemeal flour, soya milk and an ingredient called vital wheat gluten (regular flour with the starch removed) come together to make a chewy, nutty loaf absolutely packed full of plant-based protein. It also freezes beautifully. I like two slices for breakfast, toasted and slathered with peanut butter.

Makes: 2 loaves
Equipment: large bowl, clear film (plastic wrap), electric stand mixer fitted with a dough hook (optional), 2 30 x 13 x 7.5cm/12 x 5 x 3in loaf tins (pans), pastry brush (optional), bread knife, wire rack
Prep time: 25 minutes, plus overnight resting and 6½–7½ hours rising
Cooking time: 1 hour

The night before:
11g/⅓oz easy-blend (rapid-rise) dried yeast
250ml/8fl oz/1 cup unsweetened soya milk
225g/8oz/2 cups dark wholemeal (whole-wheat) rye flour
80g/½ cup strong wholemeal (whole-wheat) bread flour

The next day:
225g/1½ cups vital wheat gluten (gluten flour)
150g/5oz/1¼ cups dark wholemeal (whole-wheat) rye flour
30ml/2 tbsp barley malt syrup
18g/scant ¾oz fine salt
90g/3½oz/½ cup chia seeds
oil, for greasing

SUBSTITUTE INGREDIENTS
Barley malt syrup: *black treacle or blackstrap molasses, or, less preferably, maple or agave syrup*
Chia seeds: *sesame or poppy seeds*
Dark rye flour: *wholegrain spelt flour*

1 The night before you want to bake the bread, thoroughly combine the first four ingredients in a large bowl. Cover the bowl with clear film and leave it out overnight.

2 The next morning, add all the remaining ingredients to last night's mixture, except for the chia seeds and oil. Using your hands, or with an electric stand mixer fitted with a dough hook, mix this thoroughly until a cohesive dough has formed. Add a tiny splash of water if you need to.

3 Cover again with clear film and leave to rise for 2 hours.

4 Flatten the dough and give it a quick knead to redistribute the yeast. Re-cover with clear film and leave again for 2–3 hours.

5 To shape the dough and incorporate the seeds, cut the dough in half and flatten each half into roughly a 30 x 20cm/12 x 8in rectangle. Pour half the chia seeds on to one half and the rest on to the other half. Firmly press the seeds into the dough so that they stick.

6 Roll the dough up, rolling from top to bottom along a short edge. Tuck the dough in underneath the roll and press down as you go, so it is tightly rolled. Pinch to seal at the end.

7 Oil the loaf tins, then put one rolled dough into each. Spray (or brush) the tops of the dough with a little oil and cover loosely with clear film. Leave for the final rise for 2½ hours. After 2 hours have passed, preheat the oven to 200°C/400°F/Gas 6.

8 When the loaves have finished proving and have nearly doubled in size, remove the clear film. Using a bread knife, gently make three slashes on the top of each loaf.

9 Bake the loaves for 15 minutes, then cover loosely with foil to stop the tops from burning. Turn the oven down to 180°C/350°F/Gas 4 and bake for 45 minutes more.

10 Check the loaves are done by taking one out of its tin and tapping the bottom. You should hear a hollow sound. Leave to cool for 10 minutes back in the tin, then remove to a wire rack to cool completely.

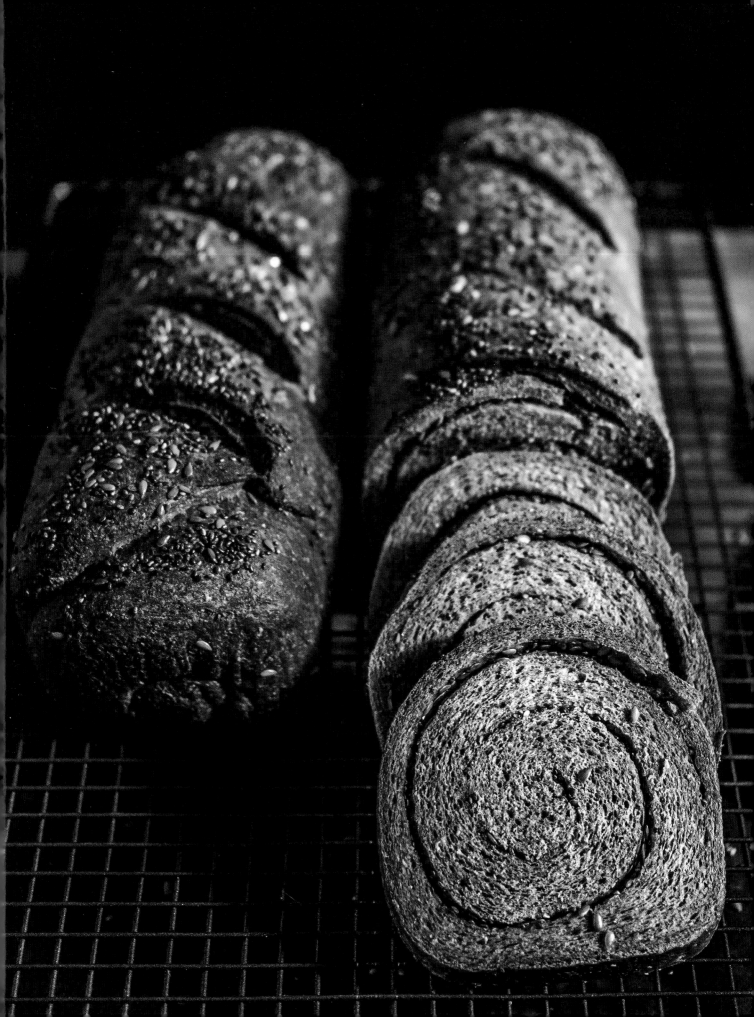

HEARTY IRISH SODA BREAD

The great advantage of soda bread is there's no rising time; that all happens as soon as the baking soda reacts with the lemon juice. This means that you can have fresh, warm bread on the table within an hour. Magic.

Makes: 1 loaf
Equipment: medium baking tray, small bowl, large bowl, large non-serrated knife, damp dish towel
Prep time: 10 minutes, plus 15 minutes thickening
Cooking time: 30 minutes

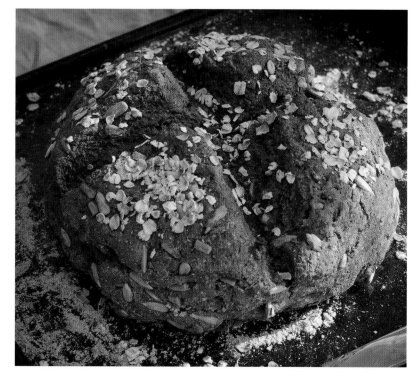

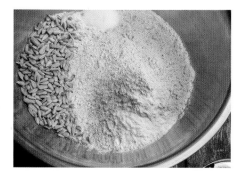

250ml/8fl oz/1 cup unsweetened soya milk
15ml/1 tbsp lemon juice
350g/12oz/3 cups wholemeal (whole-wheat) flour, plus extra for dusting
90g/3½oz/¾ cup wholegrain spelt flour
50g/2oz/⅓ cup sunflower seeds (optional)
12.5g/½oz fine salt
7.5ml/1½ tsp bicarbonate of soda (baking soda)
30ml/2 tbsp blackstrap molasses (treacle)
15ml/1 tbsp porridge oats

SUBSTITUTE INGREDIENTS
Wholegrain spelt flour: *more wholemeal (whole-wheat) flour*
Sunflower seeds: *pumpkin seeds*
Blackstrap molasses (treacle): *30ml/2 tbsp soft dark brown or muscovado sugar*

1 Mix the soya milk and lemon juice in a small bowl and set aside to thicken for 15 minutes. Preheat the oven to 190°C/375°F/Gas 5.

2 Sprinkle a medium baking tray with a little wholemeal flour. Mix the flours, sunflower seeds, salt and bicarbonate of soda in a large bowl.

3 Whisk the molasses into the thickened soya milk, then add the wet ingredients into the bowl of dry ingredients, and briefly knead the resulting dough for 20–30 seconds.

4 Form the dough into a ball and put it on the floured baking tray. Flatten it gently to form a round about 4cm/1½in thick. Make a cross in the dough by pressing two-thirds of the way down with a large knife.

5 Sprinkle the oats on top and gently press them into the dough so they don't fall off. Spray the dough with a little water and bake for 30 minutes, turning the heat down to 160°C/325°F/Gas 3 after 15 minutes.

6 Remove the loaf from the oven and leave to cool covered with a damp dish towel. This will stop the crust becoming too hard. Slice and eat.

MIDDLE EASTERN FLATBREADS

If you work quickly, you can make these in 25 minutes flat. That isn't an empty promise either; I've timed myself (which was an enjoyable challenge in itself). You now know, then, what to do if you need to stretch a curry, or turn a bowl of soup into a more filling meal.

Makes: 4 flatbreads
Equipment: large bowl, large frying pan or griddle pan, spatula, large baking tray
Prep time: 5 minutes
Cooking time: 19 minutes

100g/3¾oz/generous ¾ cup plain (all-purpose) flour
100g/3¾oz/generous ¾ cup wholemeal (whole-wheat) flour
5ml/1 tsp baking powder
5ml/1 tsp fine salt
15ml/1 tbsp cumin seeds
15ml/1 tbsp nigella seeds
neutral vegetable oil, for frying

SUBSTITUTE INGREDIENTS
Nigella seeds: *carom (ajwain) seeds, or black mustard seeds*

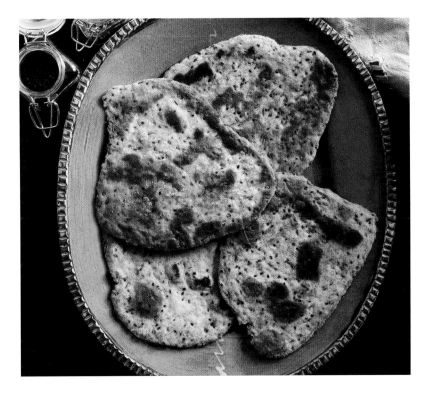

1 Preheat the oven to 180ºC/350ºF/Gas 4. Mix the flours, baking powder, cumin and nigella seeds together in a large bowl.

2 Mix in 120ml/4fl oz/½ cup water and knead for 1 minute on the work surface. Cut the dough into four equal-sized pieces, then roll them out until around 5mm/¼in thick.

3 Heat 15ml/1 tbsp of the oil in a large frying pan or griddle pan over a high heat until smoking.

4 Fry one flatbread for 1 minute on one side, then flip it with a spatula and fry for another minute on the other. Transfer to a large baking tray.

5 Fry the other flatbreads, one at a time, adding ½ tbsp extra oil to the pan if needed each time.

6 Once all the flatbreads have been fried, bake them in the oven for 5 minutes. Serve while warm.

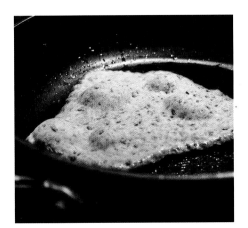

INDEX